Perfect ATTENDANCE

Being Present for Life

I0093112

✓ at work
✓ at home
✓ at school
✓ on vacation
✓ on the playing field
✓ while driving
✓ with family & friends

HARRIET STEIN

Dear Reader: This book is intended as an informational guide. The advice, strategies and techniques described herein are meant to supplement, and not be a substitute for professional medical care or treatment and may not be suitable for your situation. They should not be used to treat a serious ailment without prior consultation with a qualified health care professional. You should consult with a professional when appropriate. The reader assumes all risks associated with implementing the advice, strategies and techniques described herein. Neither the publisher nor the author shall be liable in tort or contract to the reader with respect to the subject matter of this book.

Publisher's Cataloging-in-Publication data

Names: Stein, Harriet, author.

Title: Perfect attendance : being present for life / Harriet Stein.

Description: Includes bibliographical references. | Abington, PA: Big Toe in the Water Press, 2023.

Identifiers: LCCN: 2023907091| ISBN: 979-8-9881214-0-4 (paperback) | 979-8-9881214-1-1 (ebook)

Subjects: LCSH Self-actualization (Psychology). | Mind and body. | Stress management. | Meditation. | Self-help. | BISAC BODY, MIND & SPIRIT / Mindfulness & Meditation | HEALTH & FITNESS / Work-Related Health | SELF-HELP / Self-Management / General | SELF-HELP / Personal Growth / General

Classification: LCC BF161 .S84 2023 | DDC 158.1/2

Perfect Attendance/Harriet Stein – First Edition, 2023
ISBN 979-8-9881214-0-4 (paperback)
ISBN 979-8-9881214-1-1 (ebook)

Book Cover and Interior Design by jamgd.com, Illustrations by Cicely Combs

Contents

Dedication 1

Introduction 3

Part 1: The Value of Placing a Pause 5
  Why Mindfulness Matters 5
  What Mindfulness is NOT 6
  How Memories Are Created 7
  Place a Pause: How to Bring
  Mindfulness into Your Day 10
  Children Remember 12
  Place a Pause: To Remember Someone Special 13

Part 2: Lead Your Life With Awareness 14
  Are You in 'Old' Day? 14
  Take a Moment and Look Up .15
  Mindfulness Lessons from Athletes 16
  Runner by Harriet Stein 19
  Don't Miss the Big Picture 20

Part 3: Mindfulness at Work 22
  A Strong Cup of Tea Email 23
  "I can't shut my brain down." .23
  What Thoughts Are You Carrying? 24
  Place a Pause: To Manage Worry or Nonstop Planning . .25
  No Cell Connection! What Now?! 26
  Meeting With Mindfulness 27
  Place a Pause: Mindful Meeting Tips 29

Part 4: The Mind and Body Connection 31
  Why Are You Scratching? 31
  Place a Pause: To Connect Your Mind and Body 33

You Know It's Okay to Cry? 34

Place a Pause: To Cry 36

Dis Ease = Disease 37

Place a Pause: To Boost Your Energy 39

Part 5: Nine Attitudes We Cultivate With Practice 42

Place a Pause: Your Opportunity to
Practice Mindfulness 44

Acceptance 47

The Wisdom of Perspective 48

Ghosting 49

Is it Over Yet?!!! 50

What's in Your Paper Bag? 52

Place a Pause: Your Opportunity to
Practice Mindful Eating 54

Trust 57

What if it Rains? 57

Learning Your Life's Purpose in Five Minutes 58

Unplug to Recharge 59

Mistakes Can Sometimes be Deadly 61

One Trippers 63

Place a Pause: Bringing Space to Your Day Right Now ..66

Beginner's Mind 69

A Different Perspective 70

Place a Pause: Your Opportunity to
Practice Mindful Walking 71

I Couldn't Leave it Behind 73

Place a Pause: Your Opportunity to
Practice Mindful Handwashing 75

Non-Judgment 78

Noticing Our Judging Mind With Kindness 78

Why Are We So Hard On Ourselves? 79

Place a Pause: To Appreciate Yourself (Warts and All) . .82

Words Can Hurt IF We Let Them! 83

Would You Eat Raw Onions at
Work or Judge a Person Who Did? 84

They Don't Say That Anymore? 86

Place a Pause: Time for Mindful Cooking 88

Patience 92

Our Lives Can Change in a Flash 92

Moving Through the Grief Process 94

Respond or React? 96

Change by Harriet Stein 98

Life Rarely Goes as Planned .99

Letting Go 102

You're in MY Seat! 102

Anger Soakers! 106

The Story Train 109

Blindsided in My Performance Review 112

Place a Pause: The Value of Now 114

Afraid to Touch Joy 115

Place a Pause: To See What is Under There 117

What Do You Fear? 118

I Don't Fear by Harriet Stein 119

Place a Pause: At 2:00 am When You Cannot Sleep . . .120

Non-Striving 124

The Olympics 124

Waiting and Waiting for the Response 125

The Perfect Headshot 127

Are We There Yet? 128

Do You Feel Stuck? 129

If by Rudyard Kipling 131

Generosity 134
    A Gentle Touch 134
    Coaching From the Sidelines 135
    Place a Pause: To Remember 136
    The International Incident Avoided 136
    I Froze 138
    What Worked Well? 140
    Place a Pause: How Did it Go? 141

Gratitude 144
    I Never Thought I Would Fall in Love Again 144
    One Rose at a Time 146
    No, That's Too Much Money! 149
    You Are Here to Take Care of Yourself 150
    Place a Pause: For Yourself! 151

Consider the Financial Impact 153
    Is There an ROI to Mindfulness? 153
    Are You Sick Yet? 156
    How to Live Your Dream! 158
    Testimonials from Real People 160
    Place a Pause: For a Test Drive 161

How to Make this Practice Stick! 162
    Place a Pause: During Transitions
    Throughout Your Day 163

Conclusion: I'm Too Busy to Practice 164

Acknowledgements 167

Notes 173

Connect With Harriet 175

About the Author 177

Dedication

My mother had to take a train and walk up many steep iron stairs every day to get to work. When she was only 58 years old, her commute became exhausting. She didn't know at the time that she had metastatic cancer and it was in her lungs.

One day, when she was in the hospital fighting for her life, I asked her what was on her mind. She replied, "I haven't had a sick day in over seven years, and now my record is broken."

But as her daughter, while I admired her work ethic, it was more important to me that she be present in my life. So, I placed a piece of paper on her hospital room wall that said, "Perfect attendance is being present for life, not work."

My mother never smoked, rarely drank alcohol, exercised, was at her ideal weight, and died at the age of 58.

I try very hard to practice what I teach, and yet this 'strength' as it is often called, this work ethic, is hardwired within me.

Is that 'push through at any cost' mindset hardwired within you, too?

Ironically, I was working in global health for a Fortune 50 company, and loved my position—but worked myself way too hard. At the age of 56, I was diagnosed with mononucleosis. I remember my doctor saying to me, "I've never seen anyone this old get mono." I thought it was a compliment.

Two days before my 58th birthday, I left my corporate job to focus on teaching people about the practice of mindfulness. My sister said, "You know this is a birthday gift from Mom, don't you?"

I did, and now I hope to share the gift of perfect attendance in life with all of you.

Introduction

I wrote this book as a guide to help you experience "perfect attendance" in your own life by learning the practice of mindfulness.

Have you ever walked into a room and then stood there not knowing why you went into that room?

Have you ever stood in the shower wondering if you already put conditioner on your hair, and since you couldn't remember you put the conditioner on again?

Have you ever attended a meeting at which some point you were asked to provide feedback, only you did not even recall what they had been discussing because you had let your mind wander?

If you can relate to any of these scenarios, then this book is for you. These are everyday examples we all experience at one time or another because we were not paying attention to what we were doing.

The practice of Mindfulness has provided support, and helped me navigate many challenges for more than 20 years, and I know it can help you too.

Mindfulness is the practice of paying attention, in the moment, with non-judgement.

It takes time to cultivate the nine attitudes that help integrate this practice into our daily lives, and this book is the next best thing to having me right beside you as your personal teacher or coach.

Please remember, although I am sharing a lot about the practice of Mindfulness, the *value is in practicing* the techniques in real-time. I call this, "Placing a Pause."

Throughout the book you will see invitations to "Place a Pause" to practice one of these nine attitudes. The more you practice, the easier it will become to recognize the situations when you could "place a pause" in your daily life.

I feel certain, that in no time at all, you will begin to notice a shift in how you approach the everyday stress of life. And your ability to focus will improve, since you will have the space to think, which will allow you to be more productive at work and in your personal life.

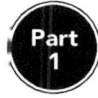

The Value of Placing a Pause

WHY MINDFULNESS MATTERS

"Mindfulness is the awareness that arises through paying attention on purpose in the present moment, nonjudgmentally....in the service of self-understanding and wisdom."
– Jon Kabat-Zinn

The practice of mindfulness enables one to become an expert in knowing oneself.

It is a way of living one's life that can be practiced anywhere at any time – while sitting at your desk, at mealtime, or as you wait for the light to change as you drive or walk down the street.

Mindfulness is not about changing who we are.

Rather, it is about *understanding* who we are and accepting ourselves with compassion.

Mindfulness is *not* about being happy.

Sure, sometimes you will notice you are happy, and a moment later you might notice you are frustrated, or tired, or relaxed.

Mindfulness is not about trying to be anything at all other than your authentic self.

That is more than enough!

As my mother used to tell me when I was a small child, and then again as a teenager, a college student, and then as a grown woman, "To climb up a ladder, we have to go one step at a time. Just take things one at a time." I never even realized until recently that she was my very first mindfulness teacher.

WHAT MINDFULNESS IS NOT

In case you were curious, in this book you will NOT be asked to light any candles or burn any incense. You will NOT be chanting and there is no discussion about anything religious.

HOW MEMORIES ARE CREATED

I was given a tour several years ago of a call center supporting the company I worked for at the time. As my manager and I were quickly escorted through the rows of people on phone calls, our host stopped to highlight a poster.

In that moment I looked down and over the shoulder of a young woman who was working at her desk. I immediately saw this piece of paper she had tacked up on the wall of her cube.

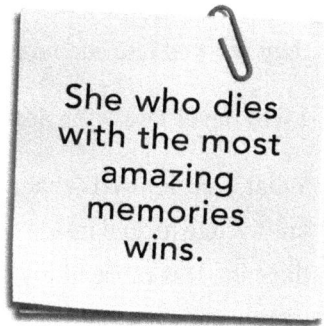

She who dies with the most amazing memories wins.

Fortunately, her call had ended, so I was able to quickly ask her, "Would you mind if I took a photo of that saying?" She smiled and allowed the photo. I thanked her and then our escort finished what they were saying, and we were led away.

Due to the limited time of the tour, I never had the opportunity to ask this young woman why she had this message tacked up on her wall. And I am purposely mentioning that she was a young woman, probably in her early twenties. Honestly, if she was in her seventies, I would not be surprised, since in my opinion the older we become it seems the more we appreciate the value of our memories.

However, why would someone so young want to be reminding herself daily of such a critically important message?

Was she close with someone who shared their regrets with her before dying? Did someone she love sadly die young without making it to a location they always wanted to visit since they were a child? Had she experienced an illness that provided her with a deep insight into the value of making memories due to how quickly our lives pass? Did she know someone who was very wealthy, and yet they never took any vacations because they worked late each day and every weekend?

I will never know the answer to any of these questions.

What I do know is that she was very fortunate to have this knowledge tucked inside her heart at such an early age, because then she was more likely to pay attention and make cherished memories.

We work hard. All of us.

I have worked in tiny office cubes, in jobs where I did not even have a desk or chair to myself, in a small, shared room with my husband and three litter boxes, and once in an office where one entire wall was a window.

That was my favorite office, because it let in so much light and because when I looked out, it faced a cemetery. Every day it subtly reminded me that no matter how long or how hard I worked, eventually that would be my destination.

None of us are getting out of this place alive. No one.

And as someone who has been a registered nurse for over 35 years, working directly with thousands of patients in hospitals, I can assure you that nobody ever says from their hospital bed, "I wish I had spent more time at work."

When someone is not feeling well, or has just been alone for a while, they are very grateful when loved ones connect with them and remind them of experiences they have shared together.

The visitor to their hospital room might say, "Remember back years ago when we went to the beach, and you dropped the pizza on your brand-new white pants?" A smile may cross the lips of the person laying in the bed, hooked up to the IV, and for a brief moment their discomfort has dissipated.

Our memories are priceless.

When we do not pay attention, we do not make the memory.

PLACE A
Pause **II**
®

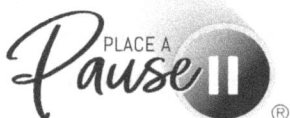

HOW TO BRING MINDFULNESS INTO YOUR DAY

You can call them helpful tips, reminders, or takeaways.

Throughout this book, I'm going to use this symbol to invite you to **Place A Pause** right in the middle of whatever you are doing.

Begin noticing all that is going on both around you and within you.

Your thoughts…your body sensations…your mood in this very moment.

Since the only moment that actually exists is this very moment…and this one…and this one…

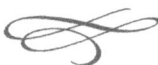

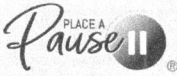

And right now, I would like to invite you to recall a cherished memory you have, one that you hold dear and will never forget. You remember where you were in so much detail.

Were you on a vacation…gathering with family or friends… spending quality time with a pet…sharing a funny experience at work with your colleagues…a graduation party…a birthday celebration…or maybe the birth of your child?

You remember this time because you were *not* on your phone scrolling. You were *not* checking email and listening with one ear.

You were fully present, and you probably had several, if not all of your senses engaged, so that you both enjoyed it thoroughly in the moment and can also recall it now.

You remember what you saw, how you felt, what you heard, and maybe even what you smelled or tasted because you were in the moment and paying attention.

You made the memory stick!

This is intentional recollecting; you are purposely in the present easily accessing a fond memory.

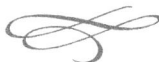

CHILDREN REMEMBER

My grandmother died when my mother was only 29 years old, so my mom knew the value of memories.

I am very grateful that no matter how tired she was from a long work week, my mom would get up at 6:00 am on a Saturday in the summer to drive my sister and me to the beach for the day, and we'd be having hamburgers and laughing in the sun by 9:30 in the morning.

My sister and I still laugh at the crazy things our mother would do to make memories with us. One New Year's Eve, she surprised us and took us out for dinner and then to the movies. The next day we went out shopping. When she pulled into the movie theater parking lot, we asked her what she was doing. She said, "I'll be right back."

My mom came out carrying two bags of popcorn because we had been too full to get them the night before. We sat together in the car and ate that salty, buttery movie popcorn together just spending time enjoying each other's company.

Little did any of us know, like her mother, she would die in her fifties. Thankfully we were able to take her back down to that exact beach, one last time before she died, and replay all those wonderful memories we had made there together. She was able to smile and know in her heart she had given us the gift of memories we would have the rest of our lives.

These little moments in our lives are not so little. But we need to make sure we experience them when they happen, so we can remember them later.

Our lives are made up of just these moments in time.

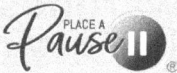

TO REMEMBER SOMEONE SPECIAL

For the next 30 seconds, with your eyes open or closed I invite you to think of someone who is very much alive and truly special in your life right now. A trusted friend…maybe your partner or spouse… a dear relative or your child.

Can you see their smile, even recall a wonderful memory you've shared together? A walk…a meal…a celebration.

With your eyes open, notice how it feels in your body at this very moment. What is your mood, having just remembered how it feels to have this person in your life?

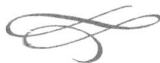

Part 2

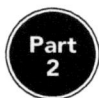

Lead Your Life With Awareness

ARE YOU IN 'OLD' DAY?

I once posted online that yesterday was challenging, so a dear friend called to check and see how I was doing the following day. They could hear the energy and excitement in my voice and asked me, "How do you do that?"

"Well," I explained, "it's a new day, and I just completed a productive meeting." Then I quoted H. G. Wells who said, "If you fell down yesterday, stand up today."

My friend replied, "I'm in old day, since you always say it's a new day."

It's a choice.

It's *your* choice.

No need to look in your rearview mirror at a past that is long gone. Worrying about the future has never proved valuable either.

Therefore, where would it be *most productive* for you to be right now?

Remembering yesterday ('old day') or focused on what you can achieve right now?

> *The **secret of change** is to focus all of your energy not*
> *on fighting the old, but on building the new.*
> *— Socrates —*

TAKE A MOMENT AND LOOK UP

I once had an audience member share this story during one of my programs.

> I remember a time when my son was playing soccer and he came off the field and asked me to put the phone down and just watch the game. He said, "You're here to watch me!" "As a mom, that struck me, but I also realized I should employ this in other areas of my life."

Please do not let the phone rob you of the life you deserve to live and the memories you deserve to make.

It's not just children who are addicted to their phones.

Your phone will never notify you about the look of disappointment on your child's face, your friend's, or your coworker's face while you were reading a text instead of paying attention to them.

MINDFULNESS LESSONS FROM ATHLETES

Every time another sports star or beloved coach mentions that mindfulness is the key to their success, my husband will share the article with me or play the video he has saved. It happens a lot.

If you are a fan of baseball, you may have noticed more batters at the plate, taking a pause before entering the batter's box, and this is because hitting instructors are now teaching the batters the importance of focusing on the present moment.

You may also see this pause when an athlete is at the foul line, or when a golfer is about to make a putt that could secure a victory. I was already aware of the impact Phil Jackson had made. He had won eleven NBA championships, the most in NBA history and written a book revealing how he taught his teams mindfulness over the years. His players, like Michael Jordan and Kobe Bryant, all shared how this practice had positively impacted their playing and their lives on and off the court.

When Pete Carroll, the head coach of the Seattle Seahawks, was asked what he believes helped his team win the Super Bowl. Carroll shared that his players participate in meditation which he believes is integral for the success of the entire team. He purposely makes his practices chaotic, filling them with loud music and a lot of activity. He does this so his players learn to become highly aware when they are faced with various distractions and stress on and off the field.

Maybe you can relate to a hectic work environment, a chaotic home environment, or both?

Carroll's philosophy is that if players can learn to quiet their minds in a chaotic environment, they can have success no matter the odds during game-time.[1]

In 2021, Phil Mickelson became the oldest player to ever win a PGA Championship. When asked by reporters what contributed to his success, he explained that he had begun practicing mindfulness. He wanted to experience more focus during his game and quiet his mind.

Yes, quieting the mind was important to him as well. His practice enabled him to be more present and keep his mind from jumping ahead as he was playing.[2]

J.J. McCarthy is the University of Michigan quarterback who led the Michigan Wolverines football team to an undefeated season in 2022 and a berth in the College Football Playoff National Championship. He said, "Calming yourself is priority number one, you have to lay that foundation!" "Once I found the dramatic impact it made on my everyday life, it was something I just couldn't give up. When I was in high school, that's when I really started getting into mindfulness."[3]

How does Serena Williams relax? "It's a lot easier now because I can just watch my baby," Williams says. "It really helps me to focus on her and focus on the moment and not think about anything else. And I purposely do that with her because I know that I just need to shut off."[4]

I doubt there is any major league sports team that hasn't introduced this practice to their Players in some way, because it works to increase their performance and decrease their stress.

Just like these athletes, what if you paused before that next important meeting with your manager or before speaking to your spouse, child, or parents to stay focused on what you wanted to say?

You would improve your personal and professional relationships and become more focused on accomplishing your goals.

What if you took a pause before that next important meeting with your manager? If you took a pause before speaking to your spouse, child, or parents, and then having a conversation?

Wouldn't it benefit you to learn how to keep your eye on the ball at all times? To harness the ability to stay focused to accomplish your goals?

To learn how to get the most out of this moment, or this meeting, without jumping ahead in your mind? You too can improve your game, no matter what you participate in.

It may not be as dramatic as winning the Super Bowl, but the results surely can be!

RUNNER BY HARRIET STEIN

Silent and strong as she pounds, the cement
　At her heels,
Feeling alive and free
　Not running away but to
That end result.

Trying so hard to remain
　Steady, calm and yet the energy
Streams thru the body
　Like cold water on a burning hot forehead.
Quenching the thirst
　For accomplishment.

Swiftly moving towards one's self.
　Straightening out the tight,
Wrapped coil of the mind,
　Body…Soul.

The pounding on the legs,
　In the heart.
Awakens the belief,
　The possibility, the dream.
A hope. To reach out and touch,
　And finally, be able to
Understand what was felt.

DON'T MISS THE BIG PICTURE

Do you see life through a filter?

I visited my great aunt in California for the first time when I was 16 years old. I was so excited! I had my first camera and took lots of pictures. Yes, I said camera—since smartphones weren't even invented yet.

At one point my great aunt came up behind me and said, "If you're always looking at life through a lens, you're going to miss it. The camera distorts what you see."

Being a teenager, I listened respectfully, put down my camera for a few minutes and looked at the view of the hillside off her deck. And then I returned to taking photos.

And yet her words remain with me to this day. By putting down the camera and really listening to her, I received her message loud and clear, and I remembered it.

In those few minutes standing on her beautiful redwood deck in Silver Lake, without even realizing it I had taken a mental photo of the hill outside. I remember the expansive view dotted with only a few homes back then, the quiet cool breeze on my neck, her humming bird feeder, the sounds of passing cars in the distance. I treasure that moment, and I'm grateful I have it, particularly since it has been over 30 years now since she passed away. And that nearly empty mountainside in California? It's now filled with hundreds of homes.

We all want to remember our special moments and celebrations with photos.

As my great aunt did with me, I also invite you to put the camera (phone) down.

Listen for the laughter and comments of those you are with. Smell and taste the food. Look into the eyes of those who are speaking.

I promise these memories will stay with you in a more meaningful way, even if you don't have a photo to show for them.

Part 3

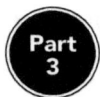

Mindfulness at Work

"Between stimulus and response there is a space. In that space is our power to choose our response. In our response lies our growth and our freedom."
— *Viktor E. Frankl* —

A colleague who participated in my 30-minute mindfulness lunch program told me how she received an email at the same time as her colleague with a last-minute request from their manager.

Her co-worker was not a participant in my mindfulness program. My colleague sat quietly and listened as her co-worker became very upset regarding this last-minute request. But my colleague recalled that she just paused, choosing to respond instead of reacting.

Both colleagues knew their manager's request would take top priority and involve juggling their work responsibilities to make sure everything would get completed on time. And yet one calmly acknowledged the request, and one experienced a lot of unnecessary tension within their body.

Practicing mindfulness gives us the ability to choose to respond rather than react.

A STRONG CUP OF TEA EMAIL

Have you ever opened your email and saw across a message from someone whose tone was either critical, angry, or accusatory?

A colleague who works in the UK, shared with me that when he receives an email like that, he pauses before responding, gets up and makes himself a strong cup of tea. He labels this a 'cuppa email' which is a slang word and originated from the phrase 'cup of tea.'

I invite you to notice what happens the next time you receive a text or email that may sound a bit confrontational.

"I CAN'T SHUT MY BRAIN DOWN."

I hear statements like these frequently when I am teaching a mindfulness program: "I can't practice mindfulness, because I'm the type of person who has a lot of thoughts going on in my head. I can't shut my brain down."

Some may think mindfulness has to do with having an empty mind or that to achieve mindfulness one must try to quiet the mind. I've even heard someone describe mindfulness as "shutting down the brain." No, that would make one brain dead. When there is no activity in the brain, that is death, not mindfulness.

So, what do we consider the type of person who notices all the thoughts going on in their head? Well, I call that kind of person a human being!

We have many thoughts going on in our minds. Mindfulness is about being aware of our thoughts and focusing on what is going on in the moment, not being distracted and lost in thought.

When you can focus on a project you need to complete, and everyone knows not to bother you. You can get a lot accomplished in a very short amount of time.

But when the notifications on our phones are continually going off, and the thoughts in our heads are non-stop, it is tough to do our best work.

I'm going to remind you throughout this book that mindfulness is a practice.

One of my favorite mindfulness quotes is: "Do not expect anything to change, and do not be surprised when everything does." I know you will be surprised how quickly and easily practicing mindfulness will impact your life.

WHAT THOUGHTS ARE YOU CARRYING?

I've heard it said that "the heaviest burdens we carry are the thoughts in our head."

Have you ever found yourself waking up in the morning and your mind is racing before you even check the time? Maybe it's a worry, quickly followed by a to-do list. Or excitement for a special day—perhaps the beginning of vacation or a long-awaited reunion with family or friends. Or perhaps you are even reeling with gratitude that it's the weekend and not a weekday.

The thing is, we are the ones who choose where to place our attention. We decide what to carry and for how long to carry it.

I'll never forget when a woman who had participated in one of my programs said, "I did what you suggested last week and paid attention to my walk between buildings. I never even noticed there was a bench there before! So, I sat down and enjoyed the beautiful weather before going back inside to work."

Why not see how it feels to let go of some of the thoughts you might be carrying around as you go through your day and focus on your surroundings?

It's amazing to notice what you might be missing.

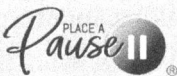

TO MANAGE WORRY OR NONSTOP PLANNING

I invite you to begin noticing your thoughts by simply Placing a Pause during your day.

Are they about a past situation that can never be changed, or a future worry that may or may not even happen? Or maybe it's a cherished memory you hold dear, a memory you were able to make because you were present for the experience rather than lost in thought.

If you notice your mind is constantly scrolling through a never-ending "to-do" list, try writing your "to-do" list down so you can focus on the task at hand."

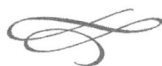

NO CELL CONNECTION! WHAT NOW?!

It took more than five years for my sister and me to get away for a weekend. Thankfully, we finally managed to get away to the mountains, but when we arrived, there was no internet connection.

No news. No social media. No email.

Studies show that the more time spent thinking about work outside the office[5], the less able you are to recover from it.

Moreover, the mere presence of your phone[6] can create distraction and hinder detachment during non-work time, which is essential for recovery and health.

How ironic! Now that my phone was useless, it was apparently working to my benefit!

Each day, for more than four hours, I sat and looked at the lake. Noticing the sunlight reflecting off the water. Hearing the sounds all around me. Acknowledging adults softly talking, children laughing, babies crying. Breathing in the fresh air. Smelling the scent of the warm grass. Feeling my body at rest in the chair. Watching as an otter peacefully passed by.

Nature is restorative.

Quiet is restorative.

It's true practicing living moment-by-moment for even just a few minutes each day will help you recover from the work stress (or life stress) you may be experiencing.

And there are many ways to take a few minutes for yourself, even if you cannot get away to the mountains or beach for a weekend. You can walk outside and explore nature, put on some music, or relish the silence as you wander through the exhibits at Venice's magnificent Palazzo Mora[7] in a virtual tour presented by the European Cultural Centre.

Make *this moment* count since it is the only one that actually exists!

MEETING WITH MINDFULNESS

Have you ever started a meeting and ten minutes after you begin your presentation a decision-maker appears, and asks you to repeat everything you had already addressed?

Some of our colleagues talk over us, some whisper to the person sitting next to them, some are busy looking at their phones or writing an email during our meetings. Some roll their eyes, some are focused on what they are eating (loudly), some forget to mute their phone first and scold their children, yell at their partner, pass gas, belch, or go to the bathroom.

If you are smiling, then you are not the only one who has witnessed these events, and might just be the person who initiated them.

A colleague once shared with me that during their weekly global meeting with many team members calling in from around the world, that all of a sudden, they began hearing someone very loudly snoring. What would you do if you were leading that meeting? Would you begin judging them harshly? What would your mood be? Frustration, anger, impatience? Would you wake them?

Would you think differently if you knew they had a new baby in their home, or were not feeling well, or were acting as a caregiver for a relative? Maybe they were just up late watching a movie and planned poorly. Here's the thing. *We do not know.*

And snoring is just sound. And yet hearing a sound when we are in a meeting has caused many a fight (trust me on that). What did they do? They determined which participant was snoring and kindly muted their line.

Daily we have opportunities to practice mindfulness, to cultivate Patience and Non-Judgment along with the other attitudes. The good news is that this is a new fresh moment, right now.

And now you have a practice that you can bring right into your next meeting, either publicly to share with your colleagues or privately to keep yourself focused.

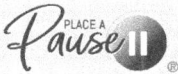

MINDFUL MEETING TIPS

Approach each meeting with a Beginner's Mind:

Bring fresh eyes and an open mind—even (or especially) to recurring meetings where you know all the participants.

Notice if you are judging the content of the meeting and the people who are a part of it (including yourself). If you are, see if you can bring forth some patience and let go of judgment.

If you are leading the meeting, invite the attendees to pause for 30 or 60 seconds to check in with themselves at the beginning and again near the end of your time together to ensure everyone is still present.

Prior to the start of every meeting:
Pause to check in and see where your mind is.

Are you still possibly reliving your last meeting or an email you sent earlier in the day? Are you still pondering the task you were just working on?

Are you thinking about issues you must address after this meeting? If so, with kindness toward yourself, remember you are in this present moment and put the other thoughts aside.

Check in with how it feels in your body.

If you moved quickly from one location to another, do you notice any 'travel energy?' Are you breathing a bit faster, or is your heart rate increased?

Simply notice your body sensations and do not wish them to be any different than how you find them.

When you call into a teleconference:
Remove distractions around you, such as closing any unnecessary programs on your computer or phone. Notice the urge you may have to surf the web.

Recognize, but do not chastise yourself, when your mind wanders to a past you cannot change or a future that has yet to unfold.

EXTRA CREDIT
I invite you to bring these same tips to your next family gathering or when meeting up with friends!

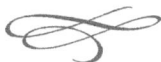

Part 4

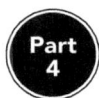

The Mind and Body Connection

WHY ARE YOU SCRATCHING?

I was sitting in my office very early one morning when a colleague walked by scratching her arms very harshly, so I asked her what was going on.

She replied, "I was awake all night. I just couldn't stop scratching."

I could see the exhaustion on her face, as well as the red streaks and scratches on her arms. I invited her into my office and had her take a seat. I asked her how she was doing, and she mentioned a lot of challenges she was having with a high-school-age grandchild living with her.

Since she had attended a weekly 30-minute mindfulness program with me in the past, I invited her to just take a few minutes and practice with me. I got up, closed my door, and led her through a sitting meditation that lasted five minutes. When I invited her to open her eyes, I asked, "What do you notice?"

"Nothing," she replied. "I don't notice anything at all."

"Really?" I said, "You no longer seem to be scratching."

"Wow," she said in amazement.

When she first entered my office, I could sense that the stress of worrying about her grandchild was repeatedly playing in her mind during the day and all through the night.

As a teacher I wanted to find a way for her to see the link between her mind and body. By sitting for just a few minutes and focusing on her breath, she wasn't worrying about her grandchild.

It did not take creams, lotions, or gels to quickly relieve her itching. It only took a moment to break the cycle. She was able to bring awareness to the cause of her itching once she let go of the worrying and returned to work feeling much more comfortable.

In this situation, when her stress was alleviated, the itching ceased.

Naturally, this is not always the case. But when other sources have been eliminated, like an allergic reaction or even a few mosquitoes that found their way inside, it is useful to mindfully consider if other circumstances are related to a stress response in our physical body.

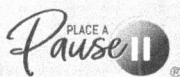

TO CONNECT YOUR MIND AND BODY

What thought or story is causing you to metaphorically scratch? With my colleague it was itching related to stress about her grandchild. However, for you it could be another physical manifestation like a migraine, back pain, or skin or GI disorders.

When you're playing something repeatedly in your mind, like, a past regret or a future worry, do you know how your body reacts to stress?

I invite you to place a pause frequently during your day to check in with yourself, to bring awareness to what you are thinking and how you are feeling. If you notice your body is calling out to you with an ache, pain or itch, move toward the sensation and not away from it.

Breathe in and around the area that is asking for a bit of attention.

Mindfulness is a practice, so give yourself some time to get to really know yourself in a different way, beginning right now, bringing compassion and understanding to what you learn.

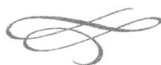

YOU KNOW IT'S OKAY TO CRY?

When Joe was assigned to me as a patient, I was initially going to refuse because I was scared.

Joe, an auto mechanic, had been working under his car fixing his radiator. He was familiar with this job, with this car, and with the service that needed to be done. He knew if he turned his wrench a full turn, the contents of the radiator would spill out. He knew he only had to nudge it a tiny bit.

One day when Joe was under his car, working on his radiator, he believed he was safe. He was in familiar territory. And so, when Joe gently turned his wrench just a bit—just the amount he knew he should—to his surprise the radiator cap broke and spilled the entire burning hot contents onto his chest and arm. As a result, Joe, a large man standing over 6' 4" and easily weighing 220 pounds, suffered third degree burns on more than a third of his body. He was placed in isolation at the hospital in agonizing pain.

I was a student nurse at the time, working a summer job at my local hospital. What Joe didn't know was that something as innocuous as washing my hands with the iodine soap before I entered his room was bringing up my own painful memories. I, too, had been a victim of a serious burn.

At the age of five, I was placed in a burn unit after suffering second and third degree burns across a third of my body. While the physical scars disappeared decades ago, the emotional memory of having my burns cleaned three times each day with that iodine soap vividly remained.

Another memory I carried with me was of the kind nurses and physicians who cared for me, a small child in isolation, with a mother who was only permitted a brief visit each day.

Here I was now, assigned to Joe as his aide. I got to know Joe well as the weeks progressed. He was in his early thirties and married. One day early in his hospital stay when I entered his room, I found him pacing, his chest and arm covered in fresh white bandages. His wounds had just been cleaned and redressed.

I knew he was in great pain. I could sense it, and I could *feel* it. I could see the immense suffering on his face. It was then I decided to say something I had just been taught in school.

"Joe," I paused then continued, "You know it's okay to cry?"

He looked at me with surprise and stopped pacing. Then he just stood there, quiet for a short moment, before a couple of very quiet sounds escaped from his throat. His shoulders moved up and down. Like the hot fluid trapped in his car radiator, trying to escape, **all the pain he was experiencing also needed to be released**. And he let it happen.

Several weeks later Joe was preparing for his discharge from the hospital. He looked at me and smiled as he was getting ready to leave.

I wheeled him down to meet his wife, who was picking him up. Before he left, he stopped and looked at me for a long moment. He quietly said, "You have no idea how much your words helped me that day. I didn't even think I wanted to go on… Thank you so much."

I watched Joe and his wife walk away hand in hand. Their lives would never be the same.

Mindfulness is not about being happy. It is about being authentic.

It is about knowing it is okay to cry when we need to.

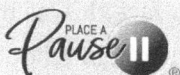

TO CRY

I invite you to feel your feelings.

Cry if you want.

Then pause and ask yourself why you are crying.

What has this moment revealed to you?

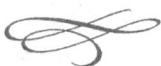

DIS EASE = DISEASE

As a nurse, I am personally driven to teach this practice because of one word that has two syllables. Disease. Dis Ease.

Disease. *Mindfulness promotes ease.*

Mindfulness is the way I have chosen to immediately provide some relief to those who are suffering in this world. I believe in the value of learning this practice. You could consider this practice another tool in your toolbox, along with choosing to eat a variety of foods, and including a bit of exercise into your day.

How healthy we are, physically, mentally, and emotionally, impacts both our professional and personal lives. And we have all experienced the impact that disease makes, the turmoil it causes, the disruption it creates in our lives.

A mindfulness practice is self-care—and *self-care is not a luxury* we can take for granted.

In May of 2019, well before the COVID-19 global pandemic took hold, the World Health Organization (WHO) stated that workplace stress was a global concern. Burnout is now an official medical diagnosis according to the WHO.

There are literally thousands of studies now about the practice of mindfulness and how it positively impacts our health and decreases our stress, which in turn boosts our immune system.

A mindfulness practice aids in the relief of pain and can even decrease our blood pressure. It is a very valuable practice considering high blood pressure, also called the silent killer, puts one at risk for heart attacks and strokes. According to the WHO, cardiovascular disease remains the number one killer of human beings on this planet.

And mindfulness helps one get a better night's sleep too, which is critically important for maintaining optimal health.

We might not be listening to our bodies, but our bodies are listening to us.

Our bodies hear what we say to them in the middle of the night when we can't sleep, and before we get out of bed in the morning, when we are in the shower, during our business meetings, and during our commute home.

By leading our lives with awareness, we can be healthier, wealthier, and wiser. We have the opportunity to be the best version of ourselves, the most productive, which will support our success in any endeavor we choose.

> *"We practice mindfulness as if our life depends on it,*
> *because our life depends on it."*
> *— Jon Kabat-Zinn —*

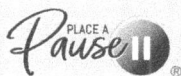

TO BOOST YOUR ENERGY

I invite you right now to stand up.

You know your body better than I do, so if I ask you to do something that is not comfortable for you, then please do not do it. Listen to your own body and make any adjustments you need. If you're not standing, then sit up a bit straighter if possible.

If it feels comfortable for you right now, just raise one arm in the air. See if you can reach for the ceiling while dropping the opposite shoulder. Notice your thoughts right now. Is there any judging going on? Notice your mood; notice the sensations in your body.

And now bringing that arm down and raising the other arm, reaching as high as you can to the ceiling. Do what feels comfortable for your body right now, dropping your opposite shoulder. Now you can lower that arm.

Move your body however it feels comfortable for you. Just for a few seconds stretching out where you need it, your back, maybe moving your hips, your neck, wherever your body is calling out to you right now that it wants a little of your attention.

And now I invite you to sit back down. What do you notice?

What are your thoughts right now? What is your mood? How does it feel in your body? Does it feel different?

I mean we didn't go outside, and we didn't change into $150 sneakers. We surely didn't put on yoga pants, and yet do you notice a difference?

What you just experienced is called a microburst. Research shows that when we get up and move for *even just two minutes*, it gives us more energy for the rest of the day!

This small practice is something we are supposed to be doing as human beings every 30 minutes.

If you are leading a meeting, and you really care about the health of your colleagues, if you want them engaged in what you are discussing, then I invite you to start leading by example and make time during your meeting for movement.

Is this something you could quickly and easily implement at your next meeting, whether you're a CEO, director, or leading your weekly departmental meeting? Whether it is in person, virtual, or hybrid?

Or are you worried about what people might think? Is that the first thought that crossed your mind? Fear? Worry? Judgment? If so, you could share the research with them. But you may not need to, since immediately when they did get up, you would be inviting them to notice how it feels.

If they felt better, wouldn't they be grateful that you were caring about their health?

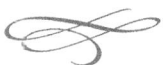

**Part
5**

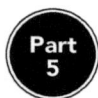

Nine Attitudes We Cultivate With Practice

The practice of mindfulness is not new. It has been around for thousands of years.

My first mindfulness teacher, Jon Kabat-Zinn, has shared that there are nine foundational attitudes which are helpful to cultivate when learning how to weave a mindfulness practice into your life.

Are there many more attitudes that could easily be added to this list? Yes, though he chose to focus on these nine.

You are already very familiar with these attitudes.

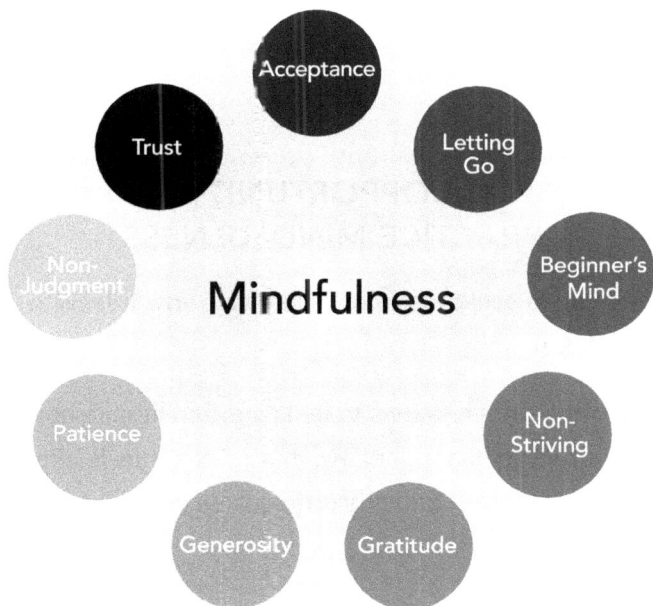

I invite you to bring these attitudes *purposefully* into your day.

There is no particular order as I review these attitudes through-out this book. I do not know which attitude you should read first today because your today is not like anyone else's today. So, I invite you to read this section in the order that resonates with you most right now.

Let's begin.

Place a Pause ⏸ ®

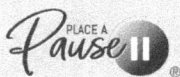

YOUR OPPORTUNITY TO
PRACTICE MINDFULNESS

I invite you to pause right now and notice how it feels to fully exhale.

Not wanting the sensations to be any different than how you find them, accept that right now, this is what it feels like to be in your body. It may be totally different ten minutes from now, or ten days from now.

You know your body better than anyone else, so do what feels right for you throughout your reading of this book.

Now, I invite you to take in a big deep breath through your nose and exhale through your mouth, sighing audibly (even a bit loudly if it feels comfortable for you), as you let the air leave your body.

See if you can do that a couple more times.

Three relaxing sighs, especially during times of stress, can produce great benefits for our bodies.

The relaxation response was identified by Dr. Herbert Benson, a cardiologist at the Harvard Medical School back in the 1970s, when he noted that a state of profound rest could be obtained by deep breathing.

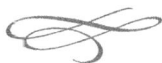

ACCEPTANCE

Acceptance

There may have been many times in your life when you struggled and wondered possibly, "How will I get through this?"

And then you did.

Maybe it was regarding a difficult work situation or an ill family member.

Maybe it involved a misunderstanding with a friend or an injury you suffered.

Maybe you were going through a global pandemic!

And maybe you thought to yourself, "Will this ever end?"

And then it did.

Acceptance is NOT about agreeing with or enabling a situation; it is acknowledging it.

You learned from that experience, and it became a part of who you are. That experience gave you the knowledge and strength to deal with today. It made you strong. It made you resilient.

Here is an insight that my sister, a therapist, has shared with me again and again.

The ONLY person we can ever change is ourselves.
We cannot, no matter how much we try or wish to, change another person.

Once we acknowledge the current situation and can accept that we are in it, then we can bring wisdom to it.

What can you accept right now?

THE WISDOM OF PERSPECTIVE

Once on the news after a terribly devasting hurricane hit Florida, I watched as a reporter approached a woman who may have been in her eighties, standing in front of her home that had been totally destroyed.

She was quietly looking at the ruins. All the memories she had made there, items she had carefully chosen... a lamp... pottery... breakable items given as gifts now shattered into tiny pieces.

The reporter asked her why she didn't seem very upset.

She smiled and replied, "Honey, I learned a long time ago, you do not grieve for anything that cannot grieve for you."

Her words were so profound that I have never forgotten them. This is Acceptance.

GHOSTING

The term 'ghosting' is used when someone stops all communication without an explanation.

I thought I was being ghosted. I was looking for a career change when a former colleague introduced me to the vice president of the company where I dreamed of working. After a brief call with the vice president, he said he would be back in touch with me.

I heard nothing. No response to my emails. No response to my voice messages. Three weeks had now gone by, and I was angry. I felt this was incredibly rude behavior. I called one last time, and to my surprise he picked up the phone!

I spoke in an uncharacteristically harsh and direct manner to him, quickly telling him how I had been waiting weeks for his follow-up as he had promised.

He very kindly listened, waited until I finished my rant, and then quietly said, "I'm sorry, I was in the cardiac intensive care unit. I had a heart attack."

I felt humiliated. I was thoroughly embarrassed, especially being a nurse myself. I apologized deeply and inquired about his health. This gentleman not only accepted my apology, he then went above and beyond and invited me to his company for an interview. I honestly don't know if that would have been my reaction to the circumstances.

On the day of the interview when I arrived, I learned he had resigned from the company, though his replacement had arranged for someone else to interview me. Incredibly, I was hired that day.

I will forever be grateful for the kindness this man showed me and the lessons I learned from him.

Now whenever I hear about someone being ghosted, I recall how what I interpreted as rudeness, was actually someone who had taken ill.

We do not have to like or dislike the experience we may be having, though it is helpful to bring in the attitude of Acceptance.

Opening ourselves to accept that the world does not run based on our ideals or timelines.

We rarely know the full picture of what anyone is going through in their life. Acceptance is an example of why a practice of compassion is so important—compassion for others and for ourselves.

IS IT OVER YET?!!!

When I ask people to share a cherished memory that they will never forget, no matter how long they live both men and women tell me it is the moment their child was born.

I have never had the experience of being in active labor, though as a nurse I was in the room where it happened. So, whether it was your own labor or even seeing it in a movie, you know what that visual looks like. The woman is very uncomfortable in a bed or pacing the floor, sweating profusely through her clothing, occasionally crying out in pain.

On more than one occasion I had a patient look me in the eye and seriously say in the middle of active labor, "I think I'm going to take a break and go home and come back tomorrow." Unfortunately, this is never an option at this point in the process. There is no leaving, as much as we may want to escape.

Usually there is a coach next to her; maybe it's her husband, or her sister, or her wife, or her girlfriend, or mother. But there's usually somebody there helping her get through this emotionally challenging and painful experience.

Imagine if that coach were to say to that person who is very uncomfortable in active labor, "You know one day a couple months from now you're going to look back and laugh about this." Or what if instead they said to her, "Remember a couple years ago when we went on vacation and how much fun we had? Remember when you dropped that pizza on your white pants?"

Just imagining these words, you realize comments like these addressing the past or future would not be helpful for that struggling woman. The coach is there for one main reason, to support their loved one by encouraging them to take one breath at a time. One. To focus on just one breath.

Any other suggestions could actually lead to bodily harm for the coach!

This is the way we get through active labor—and waiting to find out if we got accepted into the school of our dreams. This is the way we manage waiting to learn about the status of our job, and when we know, the doctor is going to call with test results. It's how we carry ourselves when we are caring for a loved one or experiencing our own health challenge.

One breath at a time.

Acceptance is NOT about agreeing with or enabling a situation; it is simply acknowledging it.

WHAT'S IN YOUR PAPER BAG?

Some of my earliest childhood memories are walking down the street from where I lived to the candy store that was literally on the same block. It was a small store with white walls, white tiled floors, bright lights, and it smelled so wonderful. All the taffy was lined up in a beautiful array of colors.

Several years ago, when I found out there was a large factory near me that sold all these old-time candies, I immediately had to visit them. The store was founded in 1899 as a peanut company, and this location dates to the 1950s with old wooden floors and small aisles. I probably spent about $15 on my first visit buying warm roasted cashews, licorice in flavors like root beer and cherry, spice drops, and chocolate covered almonds. I could go on and on.

The cashier placed all my items in a brown paper bag. I got in the car and started driving home, and I immediately opened the bag on the seat next to me, stuck my hand inside, and started eating all the incredibly delicious candies.

About five minutes later I came to a red light. I waited patiently for the light to change as I sat there with my hand going in and out of the bag trying all the different treats, when I looked over and noticed a man sitting on the curb drinking out of an identical brown paper bag.

Here I was with my own hand inside a bag at the exact same time when I looked over and saw him with a paper bag to his mouth. In that moment I realized both of us were searching for something that would never be found in a bag.

I practice paying attention to my thoughts, especially in moments when I feel the urge to reach for something to place into my mouth.

Sometimes I ask myself, "What am I really hungry for?"

How am I feeling in this moment? Tired? Angry? Bored? Happy?

Am I just frustrated with something I am experiencing? Something I heard or read?

How can I meet this moment with Acceptance instead?

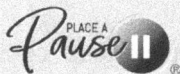

YOUR OPPORTUNITY TO PRACTICE MINDFUL EATING

This is an opportunity to utilize the attitude of Beginner's Mind from the nine attitudes listed previously, as well as Acceptance.

See how many of your senses you can engage with something as simple as a small piece of fruit.

You may have eaten this item for many years, but you have never eaten this specific piece of fruit that you just placed before yourself.

What does it look like? What does it smell like?

Accept that this is the way it is right now, and there is no need for it to be any different. What does it

feel like in your hands even before placing it in your mouth (warm…cool…dry…wet…)?

Just by holding it near your lips, is anything happening inside your mouth? Salivation maybe?

What are the sounds you notice while eating it? How does it feel in your mouth?

What does it taste like…is it fresh, sweet, a bit sour, or salty?

Maybe you notice that you are recalling a past memory while eating it?

Consider how did this piece of fruit begin its journey to your mouth.

Where was it grown, how was it harvested, and what were the many stops along the way from the field to the place where you purchased it?

Honoring the fact that hundreds of people were involved in bringing this nutritious item to you today.

The impact of so many people in supporting our lives is something we frequently overlook in the midst of our busy days.

Gratitude. Another of the nine attitudes we incorporate into our mindfulness practice, when we pause before we place the item of food into our mouths.

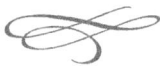

TRUST

Trust

The attitude of Trust has to do with knowing and listening to *our own wisdom* based on what we have learned and experienced.

It is also about using our voice and having the *trust in our self* to share our unique ideas with the world.

WHAT IF IT RAINS?

Do you remember a time you were worrying about, "What if it rains on my big day?" Perhaps it was an event you were planning for months or years.

Maybe your family or a friend was traveling to see you for the holidays, and you thought to yourself,

"Will they make it here safely?"

All these thoughts that run through our minds: *they are just* thoughts.

How did that event in your past turn out? If it rained, was everything ruined? Or do you remember how you made it work?

Think of all the exams you've taken. Some you did well on and some you did not. And yet here you are.

That manager or employee from years ago... Think about how their antics or attitude kept you up at night wondering what would happen, asking yourself, *how will I make it through?* And you did.

Maybe there were hours that dragged on second by second as you cared for and held your child, waiting for their fever to end. And it did.

Our broken bones heal. Our broken hearts heal. Do you remember when you didn't think it would ever get any better? And then it did. Slowly sometimes, but it did.

*You've been in this place of **not knowing** before.* And you've successfully made it out...made it through.

Can you sit with 'not knowing' just as you did so many times before in your life?

Trust.

LEARNING YOUR LIFE'S PURPOSE IN FIVE MINUTES

I once had a post go viral. It was Adam Leipzig's insightful TEDx Talk, "How to know your life purpose in 5 minutes."

I watched LinkedIn as my post began to trend. First a couple of thousand people viewed my post. Then, in the days after I posted the link, it reached almost 50,000 views. I kept asking myself, "Why have over 18 million people taken the time to click on this TEDx Talk, when there are now millions of other videos to watch?"

It didn't take me long to come up with an answer.

People want to have meaning in their lives.

Our desire for a meaningful life is there whether we are working as a technician in a lab, functioning as a human resources director, or serving as the CEO of our company.

People want to know they have taken the right road on their life's journey, that they haven't wasted their time, or ultimately their life.

The next obvious question is, how do you know when you are on the right path? Keep reading.

UNPLUG TO RECHARGE

Unplugging involves making time for a bit of quiet. To just sit and not to plan. To sit just to sit.

Non-doing.

Noticing the weight of your body evenly distributed on a solid base. Feeling the sensations where your body is making contact with the chair. Not wanting it to be any different than how you find it. And when your mind wanders, as it surely will, just escort it back to the sensations you're feeling while sitting.

Yes, this is going to require you to boldly take action in order to pause for even five minutes today to *make yourself a priority*. You need to be able to hear what may only be a whisper and trust what that voice is telling you to do next.

Even the Harvard Business Review (HBR) agrees that "The Busier You Are, the More You Need Quiet Time."[8] "'Cultivating silence,' as Hal Gregersen writes, "increase[s] your chances of encountering novel ideas and information and discerning weak signals." When we're constantly fixated on the verbal agenda—what to say next, what to write next, what to tweet next—it's tough to make room for truly different perspectives or radically new ideas. It's hard to drop into deeper modes of listening and attention. And it's in those deeper modes of attention that truly novel ideas are found."

It all comes back to paying attention to our thoughts, body sensations, and mood in a non-judgmental way. A mindfulness practice gives you the space to hear the next steps you need to take as your life quietly calls out to you.

You don't want to miss hearing it!

MISTAKES CAN SOMETIMES BE DEADLY

When I began my career as a graduate nurse, I closely followed all the rules I had been taught. Before you give any medication to a patient, check three times that the medication is the correct one and that it is the correct person you are giving it to.

On the evening shift there were four nurses, and I watched as two of them left for dinner. This meant I was responsible for giving out the evening medications.

I walked into the patient's room and asked her if she had received her meds, as there were several in her drawer that she should have received prior to dinner, and her nurse had just left. "No," she clearly responded. No one had given her any medications before dinner she assured me.

My intuition, my gut, was telling me something different. Even though the medications were in the drawer, I still had a feeling she had received them. Once again, I asked her, "Are you sure no one gave you any pills?"

She confirmed again for me, "No, I haven't had any pills for hours."

I handed her the small white paper cup filled with her heart medications and a glass of water. Later when her nurse returned from dinner, I asked her if she had given this patient her meds.

"Of course," she responded. My colleague had forgotten to sign them out.

My heart began pounding. Fear washed over me, as I explained that this meant I just double dosed her patient with her cardiac meds. I immediately checked the patient, who was still calmly sitting in her chair watching TV and finishing up her dinner.

I then made the call to her cardiologist to inform him of my error. He was appropriately furious. He instructed me to take her vital signs (blood pressure, pulse, and respirations) every 15 minutes for the next several hours.

The patient remained stable that evening, resting quietly in her room, and never experienced any adverse effects.

I was heartbroken. I had never made a medication error before. I was angry. I had not trusted my intuition. I was guilty. This mistake could have killed this woman. I was shocked. My highly competent, well-respected colleague had made this mistake. I was scared. What would this do to my reputation with this physician?

Never again in my nursing career did I make a medication error, because that night I learned an important lesson I employ to this day.

I trust my intuition.

And if I believe more information is needed, I do not move forward without first obtaining it.

Have there be times in my life when I didn't trust my inner wisdom? Yes. And every single time I have regretted it. It is now a very rare occasion when I do not trust my inner wisdom, since I know the outcome could be a matter of life or death.

ONE TRIPPERS

It was such a beautiful January morning, bright and sunny—cold, but it felt great to get out to the supermarket before the big snowstorm that was forecasted for the following day.

When I got home, I grabbed ALL the grocery bags from my trunk. After all, why make two trips when one will do? I was a 'one-tripper,' always have been. No matter how many bags are in the trunk, they are all coming inside my home in one trip.

I walked quickly up the ONE step into my house when this one-tripper tripped! And I landed hard. My arms went out to brace my fall, and my knee slammed into the concrete.

I paused. Then rather quickly, I got up because I didn't want anyone driving by to see me laying on the ground on top of my groceries. That wouldn't be pretty.

I went into the house and checked myself out. Being a nurse, I knew what to look for, and I concluded I'd probably just be a bit sore. I had finished Day 29 of my 30-day online yoga program and was feeling strong. So, I unpacked my groceries and went about the rest of my day.

By the next morning I realized I couldn't lift my left arm without help from the right one. And I could not put any pressure on the area below my knee without intense pain.

Did I ice anything? No. Did I elevate anything? No. Did I take any anti-inflammatory medication? No.

Did I continue working, having meetings, teaching mindfulness, doing laundry? *Yes.* Did I complete my 30-day online yoga program the following day? *Yes.* Denial is not just a river in Egypt.

Week #2 – I called the doctor and asked for x-rays and an appointment for an evaluation. Yes, you read that correctly; I knew what I needed prior to the exam. Good news, the x-rays were normal and showed no breaks.

And then the rest of the story... which is why it's called the '*practice* of medicine.'

After my exam, my internist told me I'd need to see an orthopedic surgeon. *Heavy sigh.* He mentioned two words I did **not** want to hear: rotator cuff. Later that afternoon the surgeon used the same two dreaded words. He ordered an MRI and told me, "Pray for it to be broken, since then it will heal. If it's torn the *only thing that will help is surgery.*"

Are you still with me? Wondering where that mindfulness practice I keep talking about comes in?

Here we go. These nine attitudes we cultivate with a mindfulness practice—Non-Judgment, Patience, Letting Go, Non-Striving, Trust, Beginner's Mind, Gratitude, and Generosity—were all in play. And one more I seem to be forgetting right now...oh right, Acceptance!

Let me show you how this worked with me.

IF I had been **patient** and not rushing (**striving**) and willing to make two trips into the house, I probably never would have fallen. No, I'm not blaming or **judging** myself, I'm just stating a fact. My visibility would have been better.

I needed to let go of wanting things to be different and accept that I had to seek medical care.

I was grateful to my family and friends who offered their support and listened to my tale of woe. To my husband who generously came over as I was getting ready for bed to help me get my arm out of my clothes. And I appreciated my sister, who thankfully is a therapist, and allowed me to cry and express my frustration without judging me or asking if I was 'using my mindfulness.'

My default, after more than 20 years of practicing, is this practice of mindfulness. Within two hours of being home after seeing the orthopedic surgeon, I trusted the inner wisdom I could now clearly hear in the silence.

Did I have the MRI? Yes, and it confirmed that I had indeed torn my rotator cuff.

I also trusted the research I found online that showed the outcome was very good without surgery, so I decided to get a second opinion and visited another orthopedic surgeon who recommended physical therapy. It has now been two years since the trip, and I have almost full range of motion in my arm, and can easily swim my laps in the pool. I'm also very grateful that I do not have any discomfort in my shoulder, arm, or knee.

I trusted my inner wisdom to do the research and trusted my body by providing it the time it needed to heal.

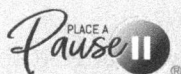

BRINGING SPACE TO YOUR DAY RIGHT NOW

Since Trust is about listening to our own voice, it is helpful to build in periods of quiet during our day so we can hear it. Once there, we can determine where to focus our attention.

If you do not have ten or fifteen minutes, how about taking five minutes for yourself right now? You are worth it!

Where is your attention right now? On a past we cannot reclaim? On a future that has yet to unfold? Or in the present with the only moment that actually exists, which is right now.

I invite you to notice how it feels to be in your body… What is your mood like right now? Noticing where your body is making contact with whatever you are sitting on, feeling your weight evenly distributed on this solid base, your weight on the back of your thighs and buttocks… Noticing any thoughts as they arise, and then escorting your attention right back to how your body feels resting in this moment… with no place to go and nothing to do. And if your mind wanders again… just notice without judgment how it feels to be sitting… maybe placing a hand on your abdomen and noticing how when you breathe your belly rises and falls. No need to change or manipulate your breathing in any way… just noticing it with a fresh curiosity as if you have never noticed it before… because you have never noticed it like this before, since this is a brand-new moment that has never appeared before.

This brief practice let you experience what non-doing feels like in your body, after all the doing.

I invite you to bring this practice of self-care into the shower or bath with you, using all of your senses as you lather up and then rinse off. Noticing when your mind begins to wander, and then escorting your attention back to either washing or rinsing.

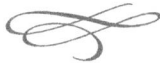

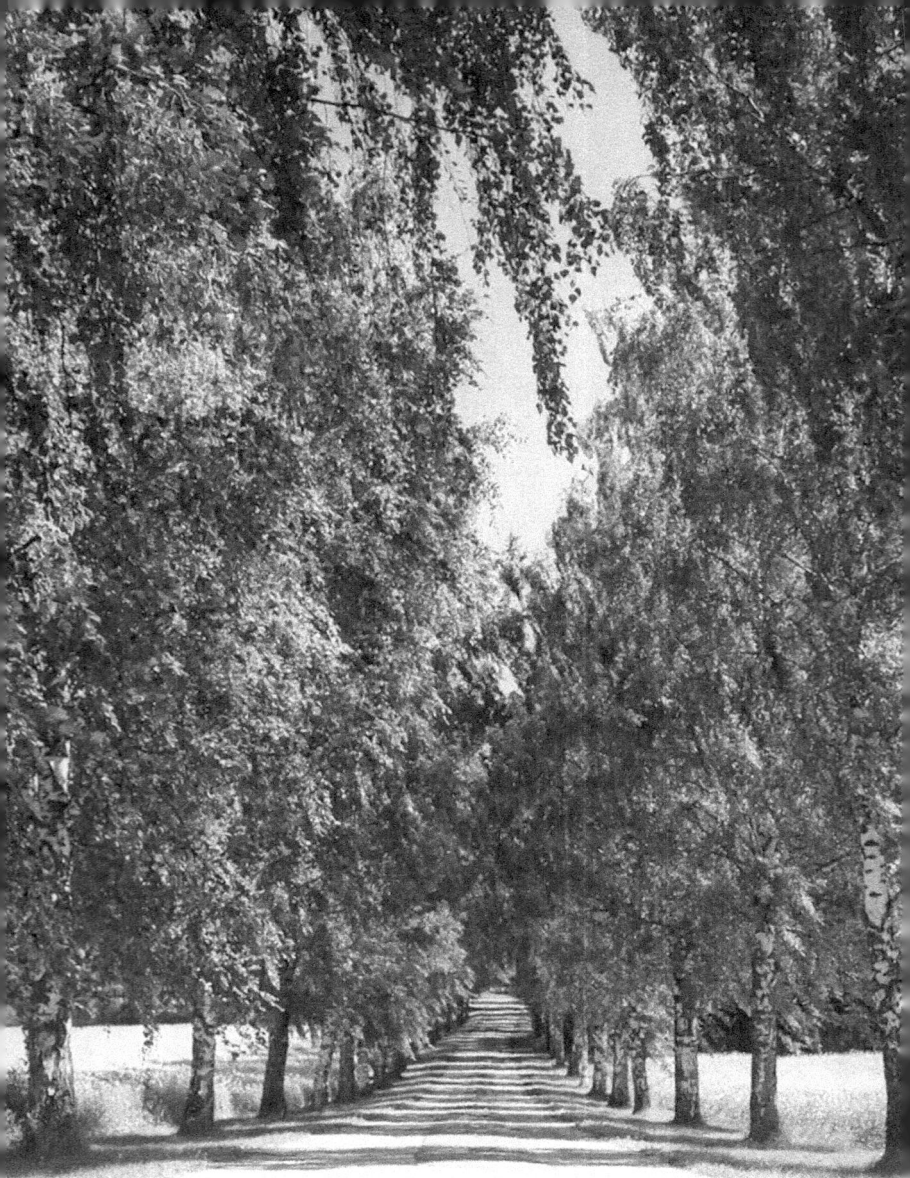

BEGINNER'S MIND

Beginner's Mind

Do you remember when you were starting out as a beginner? Being placed in the beginner's group for those who were just learning this new skill as well.

Maybe you were excited…maybe nervous… It could have been your first day at school or your first day at a new job where you did not know anyone. After a while you learned what you needed and never looked back.

Probably not too far from where you are right now, someone in a hospital is being taught how to walk after their injury or surgery as if they hadn't already been walking for many years.

With a Beginner's Mind we approach each moment with curiosity as if it has never occurred before, because this moment has never come before.

Each moment is brand new and filled with possibilities. Each hour is a new hour. And each day is fresh. A clean slate.

On Amazon's campus their founder, Jeff Bezos, has named one of their buildings, "Day One" for exactly this reason.

This day has never come before and will never come again.

A DIFFERENT PERSPECTIVE

It was the perfect autumn day.

The air was cool and crisp, the sun was bright, and only a light jacket was needed to feel comfortable outside.

I was attending a weekend mindfulness program, and the teacher invited us to go outside for the walking meditation practice.

Walking meditation is bringing your full attention to walking as if you have never walked before.

As a child, when a baby takes its first steps, people quickly grab their phone for a video and applaud, and yet you may have walked into work or even to your kitchen today—and no one said a thing. We do it without thinking about it at all.

On that particular Saturday morning, we were instructed to approach walking with 'Beginner's Mind,' bringing a sense of wonder to the practice of walking, wonder that we can do this very complex thing at all.

I was walking alone in an area covered with thousands of leaves that had recently fallen from the trees. The bright gold leaves softly crunched under each step I took. About every ten minutes I paused to notice how I was feeling in my body and check my mood, as I looked up at the blue sky on this cloudless day.

And then I paused and looked down. At that exact moment I noticed amidst all the leaves beneath my feet, a tiny little insect walking near my foot who had paused to look up at me! It was as if I had fallen into a Disney movie. Me looking down as it was looking up!

I will never forget that moment we both shared.

A few minutes later I started walking again with Beginner's Mind, slowly and carefully taking that first step.

Since then, I have carried with me a new and deep sense of responsibility.

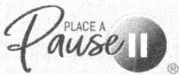

YOUR OPPORTUNITY TO PRACTICE MINDFUL WALKING

What is the first thing we do in order to walk?

We shift our weight. Slowly and purposefully, we move our weight from one leg to the other. That's it— that's walking.

Of course, if we want to go forward or backward, when we unweight one leg, we move it forward or backward. You can stand up and try it right now. Forward. Unweight. Step. Shift weight/unweight. Step. Now you're moving.

Being fully aware as your foot makes contact with the ground. Noticing the hips and legs and how they are involved in each motion. Sensing the fine adjustments that your knees need to make. Noticing the sensations in your calf muscles, in the shins, in the ankles, and the heels as each one touches the ground. Feeling the ball of your foot and even the toes.

Walking meditation can be done purposely very slowly in order to be able to truly pay attention to all the fine motor movements involved in this miracle we so frequently take for granted.

Not needing to get anywhere, realizing you are just where you are, can you be there completely for this one step? And this one step? And this one?

Walk only about 6-10 feet in one direction, then turning around, walk back the same route. The eyes are kept gazing in front of you, not at your feet, but where you are walking, so as to focus on the practice of walking and not searching to find something more interesting to rest your eyes upon.

This isn't about noticing your surroundings or expanding your vision. Rather, this meditation is about what it feels like in the body to be walking and all it entails. You are cultivating an internal observation with this practice.

What happens when you speed up slightly? What can you still notice? Moving more quickly, being slightly less precise, paying attention perhaps to the sensations of the soles of the feet as the weight shifts one to the other.

Faster still, connecting with the sense all over of walking. Faster still, can you stay connected to the sensations of walking? Perhaps the visual sensation of things moving by you are helpful.

This is a practice for anytime, any route.

Back now to slow walking... noticing what's stirred up inside of you, as you are connecting now to the precise movements of walking.

*Mindful Walking instructions kindly provided by Donald McCown.

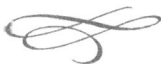

I COULDN'T LEAVE IT BEHIND

Several years ago, I had to travel to Scottsdale for business, and I stayed in a very nice, eclectic hotel. One of the first things I noticed once I checked into my room was when I went to wash my hands. I opened a packet with a little purple ball of soap.

It wasn't your typical small white nondescript miniature square bar of soap. This one was perfectly round, and had a wonderful lavender scent. After washing up, I placed the ball into the round soap dish they provided and continued on with my day.

Two days later when I was packing to head home, I noticed I couldn't leave the little purple ball of soap behind. It still looked brand new, and I just felt it would be a waste to discard it so easily. So, I dried it off with a clean hand towel and packed it in my suitcase. Once I got home, I found a small glass dish and placed it next to my kitchen sink, and then I began to notice....

Normally when I washed my hands at the kitchen sink, which I must do at least 10 or 20 times each day, I quickly squirt some soap on them, rub them together, rinse, and dry. However, now with this little purple ball, my routine was instantly changed.

I was no longer rushing. Instead, I noticed how the soap felt in my hand as I rubbed it between my palms, and then I noticed the feeling of the soap on my fingers, and the sensation of the water as I rinsed.

And then I took the time to pause and smell my hands, not something I ever do, but I wanted to gently breathe in that lovely lavender scent time and time again.

I thought I would notice the effect the little purple ball of lavender soap was having on me for a day or two, but it lasted over 2 months—and still I enjoyed something as simple as washing my hands.

I not only noticed my fingers, but also became aware of being grateful for having fingers, for being able to feel, and for being able to enjoy the soap's wonderful scent. The little purple ball of soap taught me to slow down, be grateful, and appreciate so many things I had begun to take for granted in a rush to move on to whatever was next.

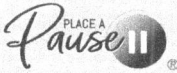

YOUR OPPORTUNITY TO
PRACTICE MINDFUL HANDWASHING

I invite you to see how many of your senses you can use with something as simple as washing your hands. How many of the nine attitudes are you aware of during this experience?

Almost one billion people around the world do not have easy access to clean water, something many of us take for granted.

Maybe begin by noticing your mood and how it feels right now to be in your body? Are you in a rush, or can you insert a bit of patience?

Are you aware of the sound of the water? The temperature as it touches your skin.

Feel the water and the sensation of adding soap to your skin. Are you judging your skin as too dry or rough, or are you wanting your hands to look and feel a certain way?

Can you accept the way your hands appear right now? That this is the soap you are using and not wanting your hands to look or feel differently or the soap to be a different scent or texture?

Noticing any thoughts as they arise. Memories of past experiences while washing your hands, or maybe thinking about buying different types of soaps and trying them as well. When you've completed washing your hands, pause and notice how it feels in your body?

What is your mood right now?

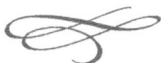

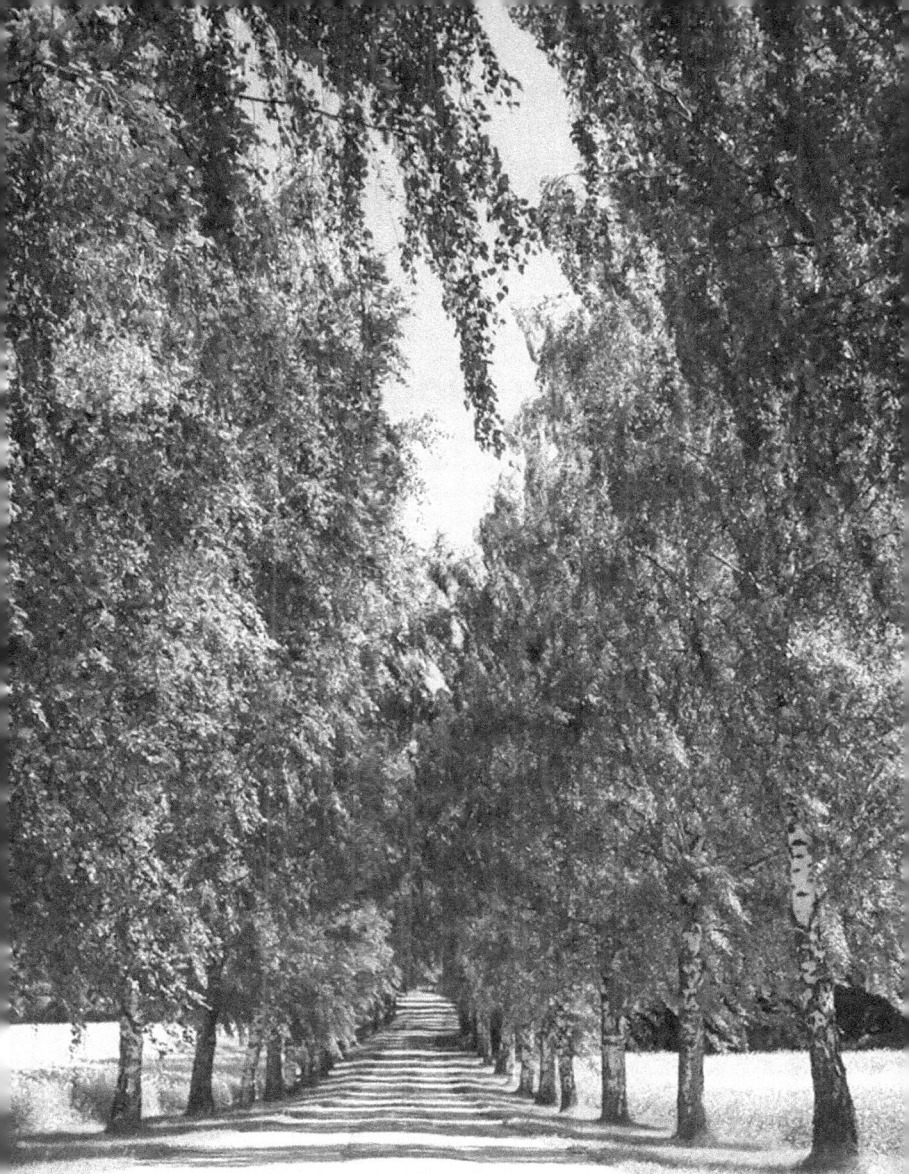

NON-JUDGMENT

Non-Judgment

NOTICING OUR JUDGING MIND WITH KINDNESS

"On numerous occasions you have stressed that we should observe without judgement—hard to do."

A friend of mine sent this comment to me as he began to experiment with his own mindfulness practice. Like any practice, the more you make the time to learn it, the easier it becomes and the better you get at it. The *practice* of mindfulness is no different.

I invite you to first begin to notice how frequently you are judging yourself. Do you remember the first time you got on a bicycle? What happened? You probably fell off. Maybe a loving parent, neighbor, relative, or friend held on to the bike and tried to help steady it for you. Then what happened the second time you got back up on that bike? You probably fell again.

Eventually after trying again and again, you found your balance and were able to ride. And even if you have not been on a bike for many years, you can still right now get on one, easily find your balance, and ride that bike.

It is exactly the same with the practice of mindfulness. When you notice you are thinking of a past event you cannot change, or worrying about a future situation that has yet to happen, in the *very moment you realize your mind has wandered, you are instantaneously back in the present.*

When we practice mindfulness, we notice again and again throughout our day the many thoughts flowing across our mind. We are not in any way chastising ourselves when we notice how frequently we wander from the present moment. I encourage you not to be so hard on yourself as you are learning this new practice, which is a practice of compassion as well.

I once heard Jon Kabat-Zinn say, "As long as you are breathing, there is more right with you than there is wrong."

WHY ARE WE SO HARD ON OURSELVES?

She was only 14 years old with big eyes and a smile full of braces. She started off a little flustered because she was late, as her teacher had technology challenges getting her onto Zoom.

She made great eye contact, sat up tall, and spoke clearly and passionately about her dreams and what she had already accomplished, having trained in dance since she was only two years old. She had excellent grades. Then she said out of the blue, **"But I don't have any self-confidence."**

What? I looked at her and explained that didn't appear to be the case. I explained all the ways she was demonstrating self-confidence.

I was volunteering to help high school students practice for future job interviews, and the administrators told me I was limited to just 10-15 minutes with each student.

The next 14-year-old young lady came onto Zoom, and sitting up straight, told me about her love of school sports (she was a part of several athletic teams), and how proud she was of being able to hold a job while in school. Then she off-handedly said, **"Though I lack self-confidence."**

What was going on here?!

I never asked either of these young ladies about their weaknesses. I don't even use that term when I interview someone. I told her how proud she should be of her accomplishments, since she just shared with me how hard it was learning her new job and how she now excels at it and really enjoys it.

Next, I met a 14-year-old young man who slumped down a bit in his chair and quietly shared his love of astronomy. He waited until I asked questions and then easily told me about himself—his love of math and how he helped his neighbor during the pandemic.

For the last interview, another 14-year-old young man appeared before me. He started off by telling me he was on the football team and how he was going to be a dentist. He communicated clearly and with purpose. I asked him about his passions, and he mentioned reading and writing. Being married to a writer, I encouraged him to keep that passion alive alongside his career aspiration of dentistry.

So, what stood out in these mock interviews with these young high school students? You've guessed it by now. Neither of the young men mentioned anything about lacking self-confidence. Did they question themselves? Maybe. Maybe not. But they never brought it up. Both young women, however, shared their feelings of self-doubt, unprompted.

The meeting I had prior to this interview session was with more than 20 female business professionals for our monthly networking group. The presenter asked a question about how comfortable the women felt on video. I watched the chat and was shocked.

- "I hate hearing my voice."
- "It's painful to hear all the *umms* when listening to myself!"
- "I look dead on some virtual platforms. At least Zoom has a filter!"

Within a matter of two hours, I heard women from ages 14 into their seventies all share how they beat themselves up with judgment.

Are men experiencing this too? I know men question themselves. I know many open and honest men who freely share their concerns, but I've never once heard them publicly say, "I lack self-confidence," or "I hate the sound of my own voice."

Starting in the 1970s and running for over thirty years, the comic strip "Cathy" by Cathy Guisewite brilliantly illustrated how modern women dealt with the 'four basic guilt groups' of life—food, love, family, and work. It was always funny and helpful to learn that so many women shared the same insecurities.

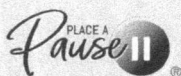

Place a **Pause** ⏸

TO APPRECIATE YOURSELF
(WARTS AND ALL)

I invite you to begin this practice right now. This practice of noticing how frequently we judge ourselves. Would we ever speak to someone we love in the same way we speak to ourselves?

Instead of being critical, try replacing those sentiments with gratitude for how you have your own strong, insightful voice.

Consider how you have effectively used your voice.

And then please share this practice of compassion with the young people in your life!

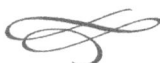

WORDS CAN HURT IF WE LET THEM!

I spoke before this large group of human resources professionals and told them how I took my new dress that I was wearing into the dry cleaner. My cleaner expressed how much she too liked the dress and asked me, "Does it come in a smaller size?"

Yes, this is how I utilize mindfulness, as evidenced by the fact that she is still alive and unharmed.

Seriously though, this did happen. People say inappropriate things all the time. And yes, I did use my mindfulness practice to pause and acknowledge how her words stung. I noticed I was embarrassed and thought to myself, *this is exactly why I joined a new gym. I am trying to be healthier and get into a smaller size too.*

Has this ever happened to you? A colleague making a simple comment or even a relative, not realizing how it could be interpreted? Sometimes people are mean spirited. Though more often than not, they are just unaware of the implications of their words.

My dry cleaner surely was not trying to hurt my feelings. So, I was able to graciously inform her that the dress comes in many sizes and where she could purchase the dress.

In 55 AD, Epictetus, a Greek philosopher said, "Remember, it is not enough to be hit or insulted to be harmed, you must believe that you are being harmed. If someone succeeds in provoking you, realize that your mind is complicit in the provocation, which is why it is essential that we not respond impulsively to impressions; take a moment before reacting, and you will find it easier to maintain control."

WOULD YOU EAT RAW ONIONS AT WORK OR JUDGE A PERSON WHO DID?

Several years ago, while working in the corporate office of a global pharmaceutical company, I went down to the cafeteria to grab something for lunch. As I stood in line waiting for my veggie burger to cook, I overheard the woman next in line order a hamburger with tomato and lettuce and RAW ONIONS. The thought of someone eating pungent raw onions in a business environment caught me off guard.

The reason for my shock is that was a rather conservative company, and this was the site of our world headquarters with powerful and influential business people. My surprise only continued when the next person in line stepped up and said, "I'll have the shrimp with rice." When the cook kindly explained that the rice wasn't part of the special that day, the worker casually replied, "That's okay. I'll fight with the cashier."

That day, my eyes were opened, and I was forced to consider old habits and business practices that were so engrained in my behavior that I had failed to realize the subtle changes in the business culture that had taken place. Instead, I noticed I had made snap judgments based on quick interactions where I had no background knowledge.

In truth, questions flashed into my head about my lunchtime observations. *How could she order raw onions at work? Why would he think it was okay to 'fight' with the cashier?*

As a teacher of mindfulness in the workplace for over 15 years at that time, I knew immediately that I needed to first pause and notice. To notice the stories, I was making up in my head. To notice how I immediately judged this young woman and man. Could it be that the woman ordering the "raw onions" planned to brush her teeth after lunch? Aren't there millions of people around the world in many different cultures who have onions (or even garlic) for lunch, and then effectively conduct business for the rest of the day without offending anyone?

And I doubt the gentleman truly planned on *fighting* with the cashier, but isn't an open and honest conversation worth the try? Or could it be that the man had a friendly and joking relationship with the cashier? Had I become too set in my ways and in my assumptions?

If it wasn't a lunch order with the questionable addition of rice, but instead a new project, wouldn't I be encouraging creativity and applauding new and bold ways of conducting business? Isn't it always worth the attempt to try to negotiate a better deal? It has been said many times, "It's better to have tried and failed, then to have never tried at all."

What are some of your thoughts regarding current business practices?

Is this boldness, or open honest communication, and does it have positive workplace implications? Questions surely worth considering.

THEY DON'T SAY THAT ANYMORE?

Recently I asked my 18-year-old relative, "Do you hear people use the word 'bummer'?" As a professional speaker, I'm very aware of how important it is to stay current with my words and examples.

They looked at me with that "Okay, Boomer" look. Uh oh. No. Not used any longer. I'm really glad I asked.

So, where does mindfulness fit in, and more specifically how does mindfulness impact our workplaces?

There are currently 'FIVE social generations' – to represent Traditionalists, Baby Boomers, Gen X, Millennials, and Gen Z in the workforce all playing nicely together, right? Or are we judging each other constantly?

Judging the words used, the clothes worn, the food eaten, the practices…the processes…

"Of course, they want it done that way, since that's how they've been doing it since 1995!" (1995 was over 28 years

ago! You wouldn't even think about using a phone that was *five years old*.)

"Of course, they just texted me and want a response in three minutes. They're a Millennial, they can't wait in line for coffee or pause at a red light without looking at their phone."

"How can you not know your WiFi password?!!" (I recall reading forty percent of Gen Zers – that's the generation born after Millennials - say that working **Wi-Fi is more important than working toilets**. Let that sink in for a moment.)

How do you feel when you're being judged?

This means to foster collaboration; I'm going to invite you *right now to begin noticing* when you are judging. And since this is a practice of compassion, notice without beating yourself up, when you're doing it. Then consider what it *feels like to be accepted* for who you are…just as you are. Ahhhhh.

Millennials are projected to make up 75% of the global workforce by 2025. We all want to be appreciated, and none of us want to be 'meh,' right?

And yes, when I looked it up, "bummer" was on the list of words that revealed I was not a millennial.

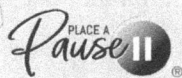

TIME FOR MINDFUL COOKING

Today I invite you to try mindful cooking.

Notice the story you might be making up in your head right this very moment. Are you immediately judging yourself or others? ("I can't do this." "They make it better than me." Or "I make it the best…")

Since mindfulness is a practice of compassion, try not to beat yourself up if you notice any judging. Relax. It's a practice, so please give yourself some time to learn it.

Whatever you are preparing in the kitchen today—whether pouring cold milk onto dry cereal or creating a three-course meal—I would like to invite you to use all your senses.

What are the colors you're seeing? Describe the colors you notice to yourself, as if you've never seen this item before in your life. Because you never have seen this item before on this day, because this day has never come before.

What do the ingredients smell like? Notice the odors without judging them as good or bad. Just notice them. Become aware if a story forms in your head around something you have smelled, perhaps triggering a memory. If this happens, then kindly escort your attention back to the present and notice the smells in the here and now.

What does everything feel like in your hands: the food, the utensils, the running water, the food packaging (notice if it is a cardboard box, plastic, or some other type of material)? Uh oh, did another story just start?

Do you hear any sounds while you're cooking? The sound of stirring or mixing or sizzling? Perhaps you hear birds singing or chirping outside? Do you hear the voices of others who may be sharing your space, or the sound of a car driving by?

Did you think I had forgotten about taste? (No worries – I haven't!)

Are you judging yourself about your cooking skills? Are you worried that it doesn't taste perfect? This is a great opportunity to practice Letting Go of those thoughts!

Today I decided to make applesauce. This involved apples and water and a little bit of cinnamon and nutmeg. No sugar needed, since it is already included in the apples.

Are you wanting to give me advice on how it could be better? Do you have thoughts one way or another on the omission of sugar? Yes, those types of thoughts quietly count as judging.

I would like to invite you instead to see if you can begin to include Acceptance into your daily life. Accepting that however you or I make it, is how today's applesauce is going to taste—and that is just fine. Practice not wanting it to be any different than how you experience it.

So, now my last question for you is: what are you mindfully cooking today?

EXTRA CREDIT

Try this same mindfulness cooking exercise with those living with you at the moment. And you can easily do this mindfulness practice virtually with others.

Just have fun!

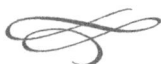

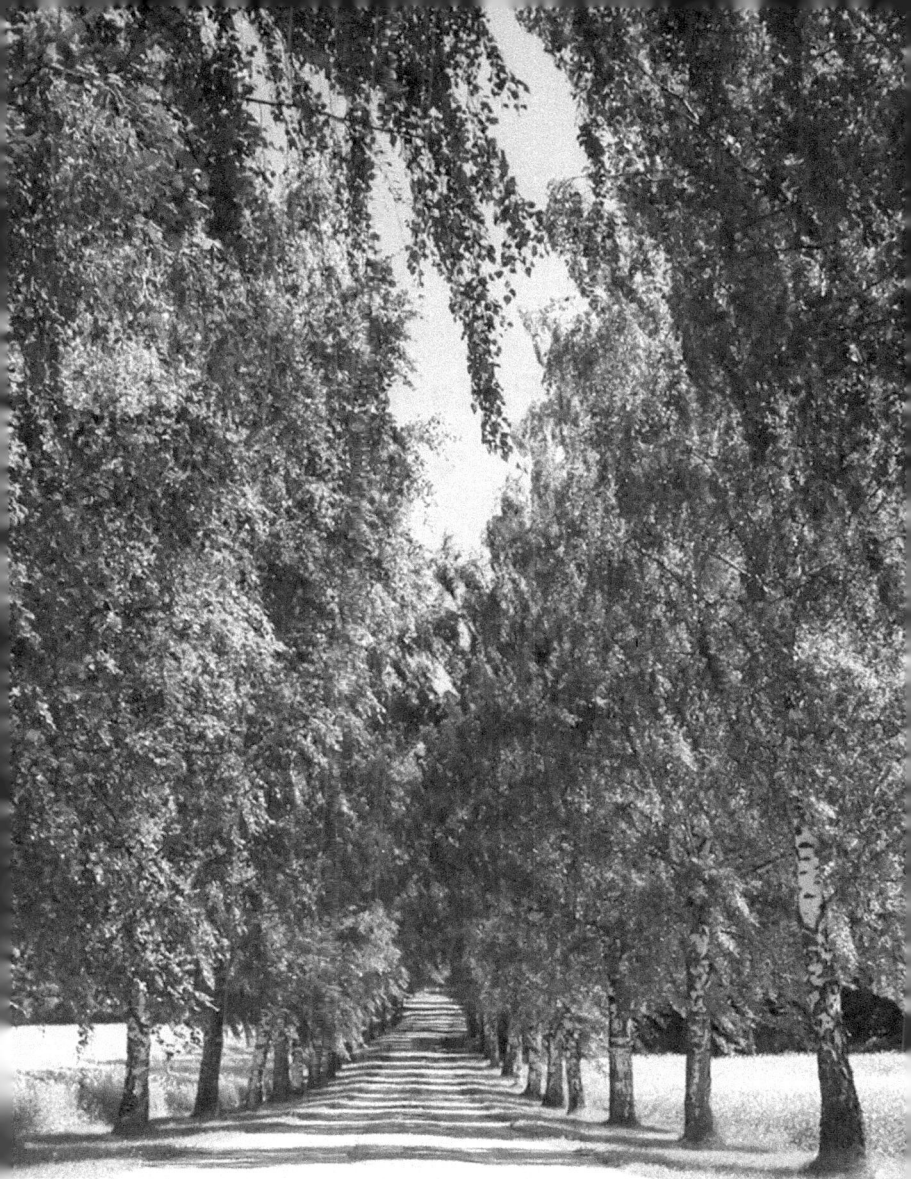

PATIENCE

Patience

Sometimes it is much easier to do something ourselves, and yet we patiently wait as a colleague reviews a project we know inside and out. Or maybe we recall watching patiently as a child slowly and carefully learns how to tie their own shoes.

We know that interrupting the process of the butterfly emerging from the chrysalis will prevent them from ever being able to fly. The butterfly must go through this process in its own time.

And yet, do we have patience for ourselves? Patience to learn this new practice called mindfulness?

OUR LIVES CAN CHANGE IN A FLASH

In just one moment.

Driving home from a morning swim at the gym, I always take a back road that winds through the woods. It's a beautiful route, but if you take it during rush hour, there's a steady stream of cars heading to work.

One morning, I was driving home on this road just after a spring rain and noticed a female deer crossing the road in front of me. I slowed—and then, since I think if there's one deer, there's probably more—I stopped my car and *paused* for a moment.

I practiced a bit of patience, even though I knew I had to quickly get home and attend to the many tasks of the day.

A few seconds later, a fawn emerged. It was still getting used to walking and was a bit unsteady on its skinny legs. It had to be just a few weeks old. Slowly and hesitantly, this baby deer crossed the slippery asphalt.

Fortunately, at the time, no other cars were coming in the opposite direction, and a police cruiser was stopped behind me. I was grateful that the officer did not get a dispatch call and need to rush around me on the narrow road.

I watched as the baby joined its mother. The mother stopped, and our eyes met. Everything had happened so fast; I breathed a sigh of relief that I had not been rushing and inadvertently hit the gas before I saw that little baby. I felt tears in my eyes.

Placing a pause can sometimes mean the difference between life and death. And now, notice how you feel by just Placing a Pause in your day.

MOVING THROUGH THE GRIEF PROCESS

Has life returned to *normal*? Will life ever return to the way it was before the COVID-19 pandemic?

People are slowly going back to their offices. There's a steady increase in cars on the road. And in- person meetings with clients are now happening frequently.

Even so, I hear this question a lot, "When will life return to the way it was?" And I think of this wonderful little book by Mary Engelbreit called Don't Look Back. The end of the book says, "*Don't look back*— you're not going that way."

It's hard not to look back, even when we don't want to go there.

The only way to get through the grief process is to *go through* the grief process.

While teaching during the pandemic, I kept highlighting an excellent article in the Harvard Business Review by Scott Berinato entitled, "That Discomfort You're Feeling Is Grief," which addresses why it's important to acknowledge your grief, learn how to manage it, and discover how to find meaning in it.

As a planet, we are still going through the grief process a few years later, and it is going to continue for quite a while.

I realized this the other day when my allergies flared up, and I ran to the store to pick up tissues. Standing alone in the middle of the afternoon in a quiet section of the store suddenly, I wanted to cry.

Everywhere I looked, the shelves were fully stocked. The tissues (the exact brand I wanted) were there waiting for me. There was an abundance of paper products, dish soap, Lysol wipes. Everything was as it should be.

A few short years ago, I stood in this very same aisle at this very same store, and the shelves were all empty. Never in my life had I experienced this.

Mindfulness is paying attention on purpose to how we feel in any given moment. It changes. And often our emotions change quickly, like a sudden breeze in the air.

Mindfulness is not about being happy.

Standing in that grocery store aisle, I wanted to cry because I remembered how scared I had been not knowing what was coming next. I felt sadness. Then I felt relief, but something had shifted within me.

Will I run into a store one day in the future to pick something up and never even think about the COVID-19 pandemic? Probably.

When you find yourself remembering how you felt during the time the world shut down, it is helpful to allow yourself to really feel the emotions you are experiencing. Mindfulness is a practice of nonjudgment, so there's no need to beat yourself up if you're feeling sad or angry or fearful. The next moment you might notice gratitude, joy, or exhaustion.

Mindfulness is a practice of compassion, and that compassion extends to ourselves.

We will move through the next phase by gently remembering that our future unfolds one moment at a time. Weaving the attitude of patience into our daily lives.

Knowing that when we do look back, we are not going that way. We are just noticing how far we have come on our life's journey to today.

RESPOND OR REACT?

When I was in college, to receive free room and board during the summer, I had to work in their cafeteria for special events and their occasional dinner theater at night.

I will be honest with you; it was rather easy work. All I had to do was show up in a clean uniform with a hairnet (ugh), and ask repeatedly to the hundreds of people standing in line, "Would you like mashed potatoes with that?" or "Would you like some coffee?"

Rudy was one of the cooks there that summer. This was the late 1970s, and he appeared as if he had just walked off a movie set from the 1950s. He was cool. He was handsome. His hair was slicked back into a pompadour (think Elvis Presley) with a pack of cigarettes rolled up in the sleeve of his t-shirt.

One day I asked him what he was going to do with the hundreds of glass dishes of multicolored Jell-O sitting on 20 racks in the walk-in freezer, leftover and uneaten by the conference attendees. Rudy explained to me they would all get poured down the sink with hot water. So, I asked him if I could take all the Jell-O back to the dorm for my friends to enjoy, and he said that would be fine.

I walked into the freezer and began pulling out the large metal rack when it tipped over, sending hundreds of glass dishes filled with multicolored Jell-O all over the walk-in freezer floor.

Everyone heard the crash.

I froze. I looked at Rudy and Rudy looked at me.

Rudy did not yell or smile.

He paused.

In that moment he knew he had a choice to either respond or react.

I offered to clean up everything immediately, but Rudy said he would handle everything. To this day, I am grateful that Rudy realized it was an accident and chose to respond and not react.

Because he responded with such kindness, I have a fond and funny memory rather than a traumatic one.

CHANGE BY HARRIET STEIN

I resist
Change.
Even knowing that what may come may be far greater a gift.

My hands are up.
My mind shut tight.
My heart frozen.

And then in the stillness
A crack.
A quiet unleashing of possibility.

My hands slowly,
Cautiously,
Chose to come down.
My mind decides to open to
Awareness.
My heart no longer pounding
Just silently beating.

Soon I realize
I am no longer resisting.
The peace
Quickly flows in and
Fills the space.
Soothing
My once frozen
Heart.

LIFE RARELY GOES AS PLANNED

Maybe you were looking forward to spending some quality time with a friend, and a problem at work usurped your time. Maybe you had planned for years to have an outdoor wedding, then it rained.

As a speaker, I spent months looking forward to a presentation I was going to deliver in-person. I was so excited, especially since for more than two years prior the majority of my programs needed to be given virtually due to the global pandemic.

Whether we needed the lesson or not, the pandemic surely gave us all the opportunity to bring more patience into our daily lives.

Two days before the live event I was notified that due to rising Covid numbers the event was now transitioning to being given virtually. As you know, there is a big difference between seeing a concert in- person and watching it on TV. I was very disappointed.

I work hard at practicing what I teach. Patience was called for in this moment. I decided to let go of my previous expectations.

I don't have a home studio, but I decided to do my best to tweak my office a bit. Working virtually for so long, then being back in-person, then virtual, then in-person... You know the drill and the emotions that go right along with it.

My husband helped me mark the carpet so I could present standing up and not step out of frame. I brought in additional lighting and got wild and crazy and downloaded a new virtual background.

I was told I would have between 30 to 35 people in attendance. Though now because it had shifted to virtual, there was the opportunity for more people to attend.

Let me explain. I don't get paid by the number of people who attend my programs. This is meaningful for me because it's why I left my job years ago to teach fulltime. I'm trying to reach as many people as possible with this life changing practice.

I was very grateful as I watched 57 people log on for my program—almost double the amount of people I would have had in-person!

Life rarely goes as planned, though sometimes it can be even better than you expected!

"The key to everything is patience. You get the chicken by hatching the egg, not by smashing it."
— Arnold H. Glasow —

LETTING GO

Letting Go

Sometimes, when we get angry or frustrated, we might notice it is challenging to let go of the thoughts surrounding the event.

When you notice you are thinking about something over and over again—in that instant—you are back in the present moment and no longer ruminating on it.

We are the ones who make the decision where to place our attention.

"Some of us think holding on makes us strong; but sometimes it is Letting Go." Hermann Hesse

YOU'RE IN MY SEAT!

I decided it was time to make my move.

I had waited patiently—a full three days after hearing Jon Kabat-Zinn, the pioneer of Mindfulness-Based Stress Reduction and co-leader of the 7-day workshop keep encouraging people to change where they were sitting.

"I will move people around," he warned, peering into the crowd of 70 workshop attendees who were all very familiar with the practice of mindfulness. "I've done that before, and I will do it again."

I turned to the person sitting next to me at the back of the room and said, "Tomorrow I'm going to do what he's suggesting, let's see what happens."

My whole life, I've been a dutiful direction-follower. I'm one of those people who arrive early to get a good seat in the front row. And yet, for this retreat, I found myself a bit intimidated by the "professional meditators" who arrived very early with their cushion, blanket, wrap or sweater, water bottle, and possibly extra socks.

After three 16-hour days into the week-long retreat, I doubted my fellow attendees would relinquish their coveted front-row seats. People had settled in. It was now cushions vs. chairs.

The next morning, I got up extra early to find a new place to sit in the beautiful large room with blonde hardwood floors.

Around 5:30 am, I walked quietly into the dark room, which was only lit by one candle.

My socks sliding across the wood floor, I found a spot very close to the front of the room and placed my cushion on the floor. After about 25 minutes, I had sunk into a deep relaxation. I could barely detect my own breathing. And then...

Tap, tap, tap. I felt as if a car siren had gone off and awakened me from a dead sleep. I noticed my heart rate shoot up, and I could feel my body tense. I kept my eyes shut even tighter and tried to ignore another human being tapping on my shoulder.

Tap, tap, tap. I opened my eyes in this room now filled with over sixty people settling in and meditating and looked at this woman who very quietly said, "You're in my spot."

"We don't have spots," I whispered.

"But I've been sitting here all week," she responded.

Suddenly, I could hear a very angry woman inside me say, "Don't make me have to hurt you, I was born in New Jersey and raised in Philadelphia!" But instead, I looked her in the eye and replied, "He (Jon) told us to move our seats, so I did." I closed my eyes once again and ignored her. I held my seat.

I could hear her slowly moving away. I was furious. I knew this would happen; this was the story I had told myself. My heart rate was now through the roof. But at that point, Jon entered the room, and our class continued in silence.

Finally, after about an hour, we moved from sitting to walking meditation. I saw an opportunity and approached Jon almost in tears and explained to him that I had followed his *specific directions* to move to the front of the room and another attendee had asked *me* to move.

Jon listened intently and then smiled and replied, "Isn't it funny how sometimes we're right back in high school? Go apologize to her."

I just stared at him, confused. I thanked him and as I walked away, trying to make sense of what he was asking me to do.

I gave up. I didn't understand it, but I respected and trusted his advice. I sought out the woman and apologized to her.

She responded by saying, "Thank you. I had been sitting there all week."

I just looked at her and said, "I wouldn't have moved if he hadn't kept instructing us to do so."

She was so happy, and I walked away feeling a bit betrayed. I rejoined the other 70 people mindfully walking outside and around the room. Noticing the sun had now risen, and our room was bathed in sunshine. I could feel the weight of my body in my legs. I took one step forward.

I wish I could say I immediately understood why Jon asked me to apologize, but I cannot. That awareness didn't even come weeks later. I'll say months, but it may have even been much longer.

If I *hadn't apologized,* Jon knew that I would have sat there *replaying the story over and over in mind* and would have totally missed the next four days of the retreat. Physically, I would have been there, but that's about it.

This is the reason why I practice and teach mindfulness. Since, as Jon always says, the *formal* practice (i.e., sitting, eating, and walking meditation) and the *informal* practice (e.g., how we choose to live our lives, paying attention on purpose, moment by moment with nonjudgment) of mindfulness just all becomes one seamless practice.

"***The real practice is your life***," says Jon.

I thought it was just a hollow apology I made in that moment, but it was not. Something had shifted. Later in the retreat, the woman stood up and explained how difficult her life was and how important this retreat had been for her.

I was finally beginning to understand the words of wisdom my grandfather shared with me many years ago, over and over again: "You can have peace, or you can be right."

Only this time, I was experiencing first-hand what that meant.

ANGER SOAKERS!

A few years ago, I was meeting my girlfriend for lunch at a newly renovated restaurant.

The shopping center that houses the restaurant was still under construction, so there were many construction workers sharing the small parking lot with those of us looking forward to having a great lunch during a busy work week. Parking spots were at a premium.

As I drove around feeling frustrated, searching desperately for a spot, I saw a truck that was parked in a way that it had needlessly taken up two spots. My anger was immediate. Because of how this driver had parked, I had to park quite a distance away from the restaurant. As I walked past this truck, I decided to take a photo.

I noticed as I took the photo the thoughts crossing my mind. I was judging this driver. I had started to make up quite a story to explain the driver's actions. The person probably purposely parked like this, since they were angry that they had to work, and others were able to enjoy the day shopping and having lunch.

Then I paused.

Maybe this worker arrived here very early in the morning to an almost empty lot and was running late because they had— stopped to kiss their sick child's head...missed a turn off because they were worried about a friend...been listening to the radio and angry about how their favorite sports team played the previous evening.

Suddenly, my mood shifted, and my anger dropped as the mindfulness kicked in. It's all about non-judgment. Mindfulness is a practice of compassion.

It's never about the other person.

It is noticing the stories we are making up in our heads. It's having compassion for ourselves, as we decide to let go of all the judging.

After I took the picture, I smiled. I felt a lightness in my body as I walked into the restaurant, and I had a wonderful meal with my friend.

I once heard it said that when we are angry, it is as if we are holding a hot coal with the *intent* of throwing it. Who is really getting burned?

I was teaching a program once when one of the attendees quietly said under her breath, "Anger soakers," which I overheard.

I asked her to explain that, and she replied, "Some people always hang on to anger and refuse to let it go, and I call them, 'Anger soakers!'"

Anger Soakers. The perfect term! Now when I notice I am frustrated, or even appropriately angry about something, I still make sure not to hold on to it for *too long*.

I know the dangers to our physical and mental health if we choose to become an anger soaker.

THE STORY TRAIN

It was the middle of the day, and the bank parking lot was *completely* empty.

Perfect! I can get in and out quickly. It's a great little break from work on this beautiful sunny afternoon.

As I leave the bank, I watch a woman drive in and back directly into my car! I think to myself, *is she trying to park on top of my car?*

She then pulls into one of the many other available spots and walks over to assess the damage. She was irritated, and she wasn't the only one.

Then, her husband gets out of the car and starts to slowly walk toward me. He says, "This was my fault. We just came from the hospital where I'm undergoing chemotherapy treatments. I'm sorry."

You can now put all the puzzle pieces together, just as I did that day.

Have you ever jumped to a conclusion or formed an opinion about a colleague or their work without knowing all the facts? We could create 1,000 different stories as to what might have been going through her mind at the time she backed into my car.

She surely had a lot on her mind. Like we all do.

Most of the time we see the end result, like a fender bender or a missed deadline at work. But we don't see the person having their chemotherapy treatment or the one who stayed up all night caring for someone who did. This is why mindfulness is a practice of compassion for others and ourselves.

When things like this happen, whether in our business or personal lives, we rarely know what is going on behind the scenes for the other person.

And what about our own behaviors. When we recognize that something feels off about ourselves, do we take the time to learn what is going on with us, the reason for our behavior? When we are most ineffective, impatient, angry, or frustrated, we could take a moment to look at what is driving that behavior.

Maybe at some point you yourself have gotten into an accident because at that moment you were distracted by thoughts of a past event that can never be changed, or a future worry or plan.

And that is how I created this image I call The Story Train. The past car cannot go anywhere, there is a hard stop. And the future car is wise to pause as well since the track does not even exist yet.

The Story Train

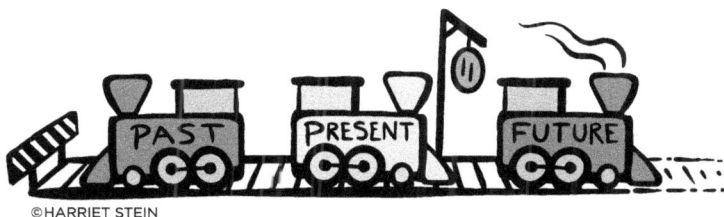

©HARRIET STEIN

As you frequently practice placing pauses during your day to check in with yourself, I invite you to begin noticing if there is a story going on in your head.

It all starts in one brief instant with a trigger: a sound, a look, a smell, a taste, a sensation, a thought.

Maybe you see a text from a colleague at work, from a family member, or your child's teacher, and you immediately jump onboard the story train.

"I already told them I'd handle this…" "I can't believe they didn't…"

"Just wait until I see them…"

Have you ever noticed yourself practicing in your head a conversation that you're going to have with somebody later in the day or next month or a few years from now?

Oh yes, that story train leaves the station every few hours, frequently every few minutes.

Beginning right now, I invite you to just play with an idea. What if you were to begin noticing your thoughts as if they were a train schedule? If you were examining a train schedule, you'd look at the various times the train is leaving and then *you would decide* which train you want to get on. If you notice you are boarding that past train or future train—simply pause and choose to focus on the present instead.

All aboard!!

BLINDSIDED IN MY PERFORMANCE REVIEW

Employees are assured they will never be blindsided during a review of their performance. Feedback is supposed to be given at the time of the occurrence when an error in judgment takes place, or a timeline is missed. This of course is true for positive feedback as well. Why wait until mid-year or the end of the year to share this good news with an employee.

It is not necessary to review all the details of what I thought comprised my very productive year, though you can imagine my shock when I received a performance review that was far below what I felt I deserved. I remember being thoroughly embarrassed and extremely angry since I had been led to believe that I had been doing a very good job that year.

Now looking back so many years later regarding this event, it is interesting what I remember. I recall spending eight hours writing a rebuttal, which I then shared with my director, my local human resources (HR) manager, our department vice president, and the global vice president of HR for the entire company (who was responsible for 150,000 employees). I mentioned I was angry, right?

Fortunately, I was not fired. I will always remember the conversation that took place with my local HR manager. She said to me, "Harriet, you're going to have to move on from this situation. I know it will be hard, and three months from now you might be blow drying your hair and you're going to think of this situation again, but eventually you're going to have to decide to let go and focus on what you can accomplish right now."

I continued to work with that director in a respectful way doing the best I possibly could, and after several months I was able to let go of the anger I had regarding this experience. I will also honestly admit that it took me many years (!) in my heart to forgive this director who I believe blindsided me that day.

When I personally witnessed the process of employee calibration that was being practiced at my company, I saw how my director had been forced to create a bell-shaped curve of her department. Even today I still believe this process is not fair, though now I understood the pressure that had been placed on my director. I'm still glad I took the actions I did. Okay, maybe writing the global VP of HR was a bit over the top. Still, I needed to learn these lessons regarding how to effectively stand up for myself in the workplace, how to let go, and even to keep quiet at times.

The concept of fairness has played a big role in my life. As a nurse I learned first-hand that life is not fair.

Sometimes people who eat right and exercise still get very sick. And occasionally we work hard and are not rewarded because of the way in which we accomplished a task. And sometimes people who are less qualified get promoted instead of us.

It will always remain our choice if and when we choose to let go of an emotion that is currently holding our attention.

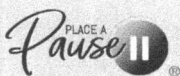

THE VALUE OF NOW

Where would it be most valuable to place your attention?

In a past refusing to let go of something that cannot be changed?

In a future planning, or is it worrying, about something that may or may not happen?

Or knowing the only moment that actually exists, is this one, right now. And this one. And this one…

Don't miss it!

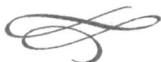

AFRAID TO TOUCH JOY

I was about four years old when I received an incredible birth-day gift. It was a swing set! I still remember the smooth metal and how hot it became in the sun.

I loved it! It had a couple of swings and a slide—and it was all mine in my big backyard. Within a matter of a few short weeks though, my life dramatically changed when my family moved to another state.

Before we left, I watched as another family came and the father took down my swing set and packed it into their car. I still remem-ber quietly standing there and watching as the car drove away. Gone was my new swing set. And gone was my big backyard, replaced at our new home by a small concrete patch of ground.

I'm sharing this memory, since I only recently realized the profound effect, this experience had on the rest of my life. It made me very cautious of fully embracing joy.

So much so, that when I quietly came down the stairs on the morning of my eighth birthday and saw the most beautiful two-wheeler bike of my dreams in royal blue, I walked right past it. Instead, I sat down on the couch and began watching TV, frequently checking out the bike from the corner of my eye.

A short time later my mother came from the kitchen into the living room to wish me happy birthday and asked if I noticed anything.

I was still afraid that something I had longed for would be taken away if I touched it. That was the story going on in my head, then and for many years later.

I decided to share these personal stories with the hopes that you too may want to explore a pattern of behavior or thinking that once served you and now may not. We cannot let go of a story and understand its valuable meaning until it has been identified.

As adults, it is much easier, from this vantage point, to look back and bring kindness to the way we responded as young children. Though, do we?

Or do we judge the patterns once we've identified them through adult eyes, forgetting that we were young children when we experienced these situations that set these patterns in place?

> *"A family's responses to crisis or to a new situation mirror those of a child.*
>
> *That is to say, the way a small child deals with a new challenge (for instance, learning to walk) has certain predictable stages: regression, anxiety, mastery, new energy, growth, and feedback for future achievement.*
>
> *These stages can also be seen in adults coping with new life events, whether positive or negative."*
>
> — T. Berry Brazelton —

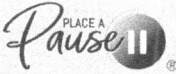

TO SEE WHAT IS UNDER THERE

I invite you take a moment to consider a behavior or mindset you may be aware of that you have had for quite a while. It could be a pattern like thinking something bad is going to happen because something good just occurred in your life. Or maybe you notice a consistent behavior such as being stubborn or impatient.

Can you see when this behavior began? Is this behavior that served you well in the past, maybe as a child, still one you want to practice in adulthood? Or could it be time to let that behavior go?

Letting Go is not about forgetting or dropping a long-held belief. Instead, the first step in Letting Go is gently excavating the stories we tell ourselves with compassion with the intention of truly understanding ourselves without judgment.

We can continue our journey through life bumping down the road, perhaps ignoring the noise we hear in the car, like the thoughts that rest in our hearts.

Or we can choose to purposefully Let Go with Gratitude for the way this experience served us in the past and appreciation for the lessons we have learned that have safely brought us to today.

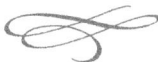

WHAT DO YOU FEAR?

Someone once asked me, "What do you fear?" It was expressed very matter-of-factly, as if this was a commonly discussed subject. But it isn't. I think about what worries me a lot, but fear, that's a whole different ball of wax.

So, I thought about it and replied, "I'm afraid I won't make it to this meditation class on time during rush hour."

"No," she replied. "What do you fear about life?"

So, I thought about it some more and replied honestly, "Nothing."

I guess nobody had ever responded to her that way before because for a moment she looked at me like I had said, "Drinking milk," or "Choking while brushing my teeth."

Then she tried plan B. "Don't you fear dying of pancreatic cancer?" (I swear this is the truth, by the way. The older I get; I'm constantly reminded how the truth is so much stranger than fiction.)

"No, I don't," I responded unable to suppress an uncomfortable smile. I knew even then how strange her question was. I now began to wonder if this was her fear.

But enough about this odd encounter. What does this all mean to me? And should I be afraid?

I DON'T FEAR BY HARRIET STEIN

That was me, over there, the scared one.

Afraid of going through life without a father. It happened. I still soared. Afraid of not making the grades I needed. I did and succeeded.

Afraid no one would ever ask me to the prom. They didn't. I asked. I went.

Afraid of living alone. What if the toilet backed up, or a wasp got in my home, or my roof leaked? They did. I survived.

Afraid of what would happen if my mother, my dear mother, ever got sick. She did. She died. I lived. Never the same, yet stronger. More compassionate.

Afraid of flying after an experience at 30,000 feet left me shaken to the core. It happened once. I've flown safely since. It's over; the skies are mine again.

Afraid of never finding a man to share my life with. I've dated. And dated. And dated. I've grown, and cried, and laughed. I've loved, and hugged, and sighed. Afraid of not finding him? No longer. Afraid he may not find me? No longer.

Afraid of loss. I've lost. Afraid of love. I've loved.

Afraid of pain. I've hurt and healed.

Afraid of living. I've lived.

There it is.

The anecdote to fear. Fearing. Knowing it. And then letting it go.

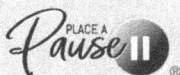

AT 2:00 AM WHEN YOU CANNOT SLEEP

Sleep is an excellent example of how you already practice the attitude of Letting Go every night.

Waking up two to three times during the night is actually a normal part of our sleep pattern. Infants can sleep six to eight hours straight throughout the night, rarely adults.

Have you ever had the experience where you wake up at 2:00 am and maybe get up and use the bathroom, then return to bed, and now you are wide awake and cannot get back to sleep?

What do you do?

If you check your phone, I will start crying right now. Please, do not check your phone.

Once you take even a quick look at your phone, you will immediately become psychologically engaged. Smartphones were specifically developed in a way to engage you, and they were quite successful in achieving their goal. The emails can wait. Social media can wait. The news can wait.

The necessity for you to get a really good night's sleep cannot wait.

I invite you to try a mindfulness practice called a body scan the next time you find yourself wide awake in the middle of the night.

Bring your attention to your body and away from the many thoughts crossing your mind.

Beginning with your feet, noticing if they are cold or if they are warm, maybe they feel damp or dry, maybe you notice the weight of a blanket or sheet on them. Maybe they feel tingly, maybe you don't feel any sensation at all, and that is fine. Not wanting your feet to be in any way different than how you find them.

And now slowly moving up your body to your calves, and then to your knees, and then to your upper legs, to your buttocks, and to your lower back.

Slowly and patiently moving up your body, just noticing the sensation in each of those body parts, noticing the temperature, noticing the weight of where they are resting upon the bed.

Maybe there is a little tightness in the knee or a little achiness in a hip, take the time to really explore these sensations instead of moving away from them.

And if you notice your mind wandering to thoughts about past events that you cannot change or a future plan, or possibly a worry, then gently escort your attention right back to what it feels like in your body.

Allowing your body to experience the rest it needs and deserves.

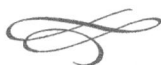

NON-STRIVING

Non-Striving

Another one of the attitudes we cultivate with a mindfulness practice is Non-Striving.

Non-Striving does not mean giving up. Rather, Non-Striving allows us to pause and notice our desire to want to make things go our way, instead of allowing them to be just as they are.

Non-Striving is realizing you are enough right now, exactly the way you are.

THE OLYMPICS

During the Olympics one year, I watched as a reporter thrust their microphone into the face of a young woman who just moments before had won her first gold medal and asked her, "So, what's next?"

Really?!

Can you even imagine the hours this Olympian had spent training since she was a young child? Rising before the sun when it was dark and cold to make her way to a training facility, and then having to go to school, and then having to train more after school. Month after month, year after year. Exhaustion. Pressure. Joy. Pride. So many emotions.

Can you imagine after spending eight hours in active labor, that seconds after your beautiful child is born, the doctor turns to you and asks, "So, when do you think you will be having another child?"

Really?!

These special moments do not need to include an award ceremony.

Maybe it is giving a great presentation, celebrating a personal achievement, or just actively listening to a loved one share treasured stories for the one hundredth time sitting around the table during the holidays and not interrupting their storytelling.

I am going to invite you to see if you can pay closer attention to the moments and allow life to unfold just as it is meant to be.

WAITING AND WAITING FOR THE RESPONSE

A friend of mine spent many weeks trying to establish a relationship with a new client. Finally, the person agreed and said they would be willing to work with them. My friend sent them a contract on Friday, which the new client said they would sign and return.

On Monday morning, my friend still had not received the completed agreement. They began to feel anxious; they wanted to e-mail or call this new client. Fortunately, they called me instead.

I invited my friend to notice all the stories that were floating around in their head about why the client hadn't immediately stopped their life to sign their agreement and quickly return it to them. This new client had a great deal of responsibility as the leader of their own company. Upon entering their business on Monday morning, they may have had to deal with several issues, possibly a few of an urgent nature.

I invited my friend to begin practicing Non-Striving. To be aware of the urge to pick up the phone or write and begin to weave in all these attitudes that are the foundation of a mindfulness practice instead.

I encouraged them to actively practice Patience, Letting Go, Trust, and Non-Striving. And yes, a bit of Non-Judgment too, if that was now entering into the picture as well.

My advice was to not in any way contact the potential new client. They listened and accepted my advice.

On Wednesday my friend called to inform me that the signed agreement arrived.

Waiting is not easy for any of us, especially when the stakes are high. Anxiety can manifest as we wait for a doctor to call with test results, or start bubbling when a manager unexpectedly requests a meeting with you alone on a Friday morning.

Being present in your life is powerful. This may bring you the peace of mind you seek. In contrast, consider what living with worry, anger, and regret does to our physical and mental health.

Remember, the only moment that actually exists is this one… right now! Be present.

THE PERFECT HEADSHOT

I once attended a very large conference. It was mentioned that certain booths in the Exhibit Hall were offering free headshots. So, during the break, I, along with 10,000 other women, quickly ran over to get in line and patiently wait for our new headshot.

After mine was taken I looked at it carefully and decided to try another booth. I actually waited in those long lines at three different booths trying so hard to get that elusive perfect headshot.

It did not happen.

I later told my friend about my quest for the perfect headshot, and he replied, "Harriet, your 'striver's license' has been revoked!" Though in actuality I think I earned it that day!

ARE WE THERE YET?

People frequently tell me, "I can't take it anymore!"

The COVID-19 global pandemic surely stretched us all to the limit, even though as I'm writing this, we are on year three of this event.

If you are beating yourself up because you have not met the performance goals you worked so hard to achieve, or in a moment of exhaustion became impatient with your child, spouse, friend, lover, pet, colleague, or stranger, then I'm going to encourage you to forgive yourself.

We are all human and doing the best we can under very difficult circumstances.

> *"We are not all in the same boat. We are all in the same storm. Some of us are on super-yachts. Some have just the one oar."*
> — *Damian Barr* —

Maybe you don't need to be concerned about paying rent, a mortgage, health insurance bills, school tuition, or a myriad of other critically important needs, but many people do. I invite you to do what you can, when you can, for others.

And if now, possibly for the first time in your entire life, you must focus on yourself, then please do what is best for you.

This attitude of Non-Striving does not mean giving up. Non-Striving allows us to pause and notice our desire to want to make things go our way instead of allowing them to be just as they are.

This pandemic will one day come to an end—history has surely shown us this. In the meantime, we will do what we can do right now. We can cultivate Patience.

We can curse the thorns, or we can appreciate the rose.

DO YOU FEEL STUCK?

Are you waiting for news on how your company will move forward or to see if your child will get accepted into their preferred school, internship, or job this year?

Maybe you're trying to schedule a vacation for the first time in a long time and having trouble finalizing trip plans. Is your contractor returning your calls? Are you waiting to hear back from a client who seemed so interested in working with you? Are you trying to determine whether to hold a meeting in person, virtually, or make it hybrid, and still waiting for insight from the decision-maker?

This 'stuck' feeling happens to us all at some point. Frustrating? Yes!

It is easy to list times from our past when we were actively striving:

- Wanting so much to make the team.

- Wishing we were taller, thinner, older, younger, or stronger.

- Praying we would get that good news—a college acceptance letter, a romantic proposal, a positive pregnancy test.

- Hoping that the fifth interview was the last and they'd realize we were perfect for the job.

Those hours, weeks or months of waiting seem like years. This is when I'm going to encourage you to cultivate the attitude of Non-Striving as part of your mindfulness practice.

When I feel a desire, an urge, to have life move faster, I take note of it.

Like you, I have been here before. I know the only thing that will bring me some relief is really embracing this practice. Actively Letting Go when I notice myself worrying about the future, remembering to Trust the process, and let things play out, and having the Patience to know that this too shall pass.

And then I read this poem I've cherished for decades that has helped me get through so many of these striving moments.

IF BY RUDYARD KIPLING

If you can keep your head when all about you
   Are losing theirs and blaming it on you,

If you can trust yourself when all men doubt you,
   But make allowance for their doubting too;

If you can wait and not be tired by waiting,
   Or being lied about, don't deal in lies,

Or being hated, don't give way to hating,
   And yet don't look too good, nor talk too wise:

If you can dream—and not make dreams your master;
   If you can think—and not make thoughts your aim;

If you can meet with Triumph and Disaster
   And treat those two impostors just the same;

If you can bear to hear the truth you've spoken
   Twisted by knaves to make a trap for fools,

Or watch the things you gave your life to, broken,
   And stoop and build 'em up with worn-out tools:

If you can make one heap of all your winnings
    And risk it on one turn of pitch-and-toss,

And lose, and start again at your beginnings
    And never breathe a word about your loss;

If you can force your heart and nerve and sinew
    To serve your turn long after they are gone,

And so hold on when there is nothing in you
    Except the will which says to them: 'Hold on!'

If you can talk with crowds and keep your virtue,
    Or walk with Kings—nor lose the common touch,

If neither foes nor loving friends can hurt you,
    If all men count with you, but none too much;

If you can fill the unforgiving minute
    With sixty seconds' worth of distance run,

Yours is the Earth and everything that's in it,
    And—which is more—you'll be a man, my son!

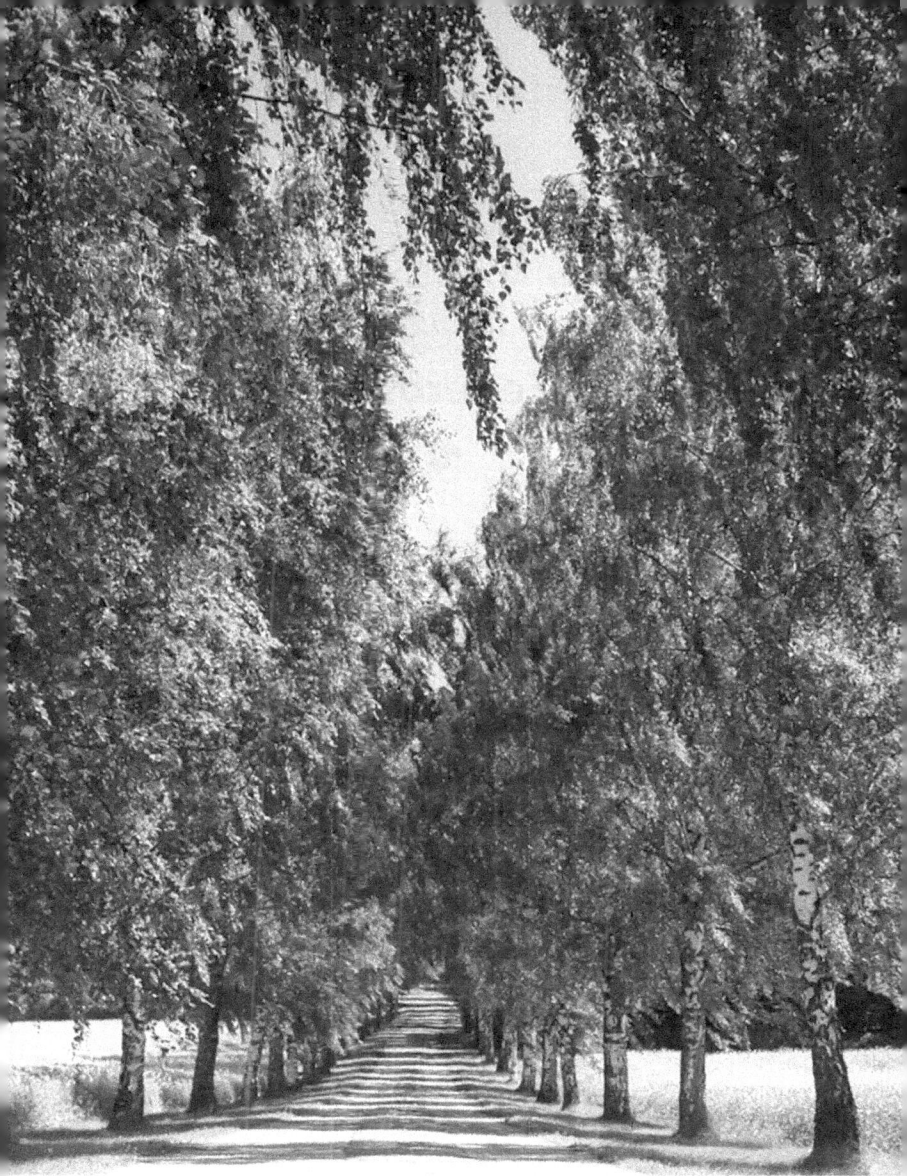

GENEROSITY

Generosity

A GENTLE TOUCH

Sitting at a stoplight a couple of years ago, I watched as an older boy quietly talked to what I am thinking may have been his younger brother. And then I watched him do something very unexpected on this busy street with so many people rushing to get to work, or drop off their children for school.

He reached out and put his arm around him.

The older brother may have been around 10 years old and the younger brother around six years old. You could write your own story as to why someone's day could start this way.

And another story about the man that older brother is going to grow up to become, based on the level of compassion he is already demonstrating.

COACHING FROM THE SIDELINES

Novak Djokovic is a professional tennis player and was ranked #1 in the world by the Association of Tennis Professionals.

In June of 2021, moments after winning the French Open, his second Grand Slam title of the year, Novak Djokovic passed off his game-winning racket to a young fan in the stands, who was ecstatic to receive such a gift. This young man literally cried tears of joy as he was jumping up and down to the delight of millions of viewers watching.

And why did Djokovic place this pause in his day as he was quickly walking off the court?

> *"I don't know the boy, but he was in my ear the entire match, especially when I was two sets down. He was encouraging me, and he was actually giving me tactics as well… **He was coaching me**, literally, and so I found that very cute and very nice. I felt like to give the racquet, the best person was him.*
>
> *That was kind of my gratitude for him for sticking with me and supporting me."*[9]

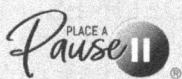

TO REMEMBER

Do you remember the last time someone at work or in your personal life expressed their generosity for something you did?

Do you recall how it made you feel?

Or maybe you were the one who was on the receiving end, as someone kindly helped you out at work or home.

Do you recall how that made you feel as the recipient?

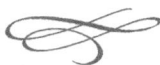

THE INTERNATIONAL INCIDENT AVOIDED

I will never forget the kindness shown to me when I was responsible for implementing a global training program.

Each participant who attended the session was provided with a beautifully designed box.

The box was made of cardboard and appeared so very expensive that a vice president expressed their anger at the cost, until it was explained to them the cost was minimal. Inside the box was a notebook with a copy of the slides being used during the presentation, a combination highlighter and pen, and a small clock.

When I asked my training colleagues in China how their session went, they informed me the attendees found the program very valuable.

I asked about the beautiful box everyone received and what they thought of the clock, and the

trainer replied, "They really liked the calendar."

Calendar? I was confused and explained that it was a clock.

My Chinese training colleague very kindly informed me that in China, giving someone a gift of a clock is considered bad luck. It would be as if you were highlighting that their time was running out!

OH, NO! I screamed inside my head. I was shocked, embarrassed, and very concerned about the mistake I had inadvertently made. I had no idea this simple gesture of a gift could be considered rude in another culture.

I learned a lot of lessons from this experience, and most importantly appreciated the generosity of how another trainer around the world immediately had my back so as to prevent me from looking foolish.

Since I was not present, I do not know how she explained away my *faux pas*, though I know how I felt when she assured me everything was okay, and no one was offended.

I was so very grateful for the generosity she exhibited toward me.

I FROZE

I was so excited to be going on my very first business trip. I had recently left a position in which I worked on a busy medical unit as a nurse, and now I was the hospital's patient advocate. I would be attending a national conference in the Midwest, and my best suit was packed.

Once I arrived at the hotel and checked into my room, I went out for a walk to familiarize myself with my new surroundings. I returned a few hours later and headed for the elevators to relax a bit in my room before dinner. The elevator doors opened, and I froze.

I wish I hadn't frozen. We spend thousands of hours in front of TV and movie screens (and now phones and tablets) looking at horrific images made to scare us...which can sometimes even numb us to the pain of others.

I was faced with a middle-aged man, his face severely affected by Neurofibromatosis (a condition *incorrectly* associated with Joseph Merrick called Elephant Man's Disease, since Merrick had Proteus syndrome). I just froze for a split-second debating on whether to enter the empty elevator with him. *And he knew that.*

I walked quickly inside, the elevator doors closed, and I was alone with this gentleman. I frantically tried to think of something to say to him to assuage my guilt and strike up a conversation to show him the compassionate person I really am versus the scared version he just witnessed. Was he attending the conference? Had he ever been to this city before? Just when I was about to speak, *he turned away from me.*

Over the next several days I looked for him and yet never saw him again. Was he the husband of a conference attendee? I'll never know. I lost an opportunity to show compassion and in the blink of an eye my chance was gone forever.

As a nurse I cared for so many patients with a multitude of challenges, treating them all with compassion and dignity. Old or young, male or female, they were all humans just wanting to be free of pain and embarrassment. They yearned for health and happiness and respect.

I never looked away because everyone deserves to be seen.

The missed opportunity of showing a fellow traveler respect reminds me of how important it is to never become numb to someone else's pain and suffering, and always demonstrate compassion with each opportunity as it unexpectedly arises.

WHAT WORKED WELL?

In 2014 I read an article entitled, "People would rather be electrically shocked than left alone with their thoughts," posted in Science10.

Those of us who teach the practice of mindfulness are very aware of this challenge. It is why we must first embody this practice before we can share it with anyone.

I spent years in training to be an advanced mindfulness teacher learning what to say, what not to say, and when to hold my seat and my tongue. I was very fortunate to learn from the two teachers who actually wrote the first practical guide for clinicians and educators, Donald McCown and Diane Reibel.

Finally, the time came for me to teach my first solo program. Even though at least 15 years have now passed, I remember my concerns very well. I felt as if I was holding the hearts of every attendee in my hands during that first two-hour program.

After delivering the program I met with Don, who knew I was very nervous. He inquired as to how I thought it went from my perspective.

I excitedly began, "I forgot to mention…I wish I would have…"

Don stopped me.

"Harriet," he asked, "Tell me first what went right?"

That simple instruction changed everything for me, in both my professional and personal life, from that very moment forward.

How often when someone asks you, "How did your meeting go…how was that event you hosted…how are you doing?" Do you lead with the negative? All those judgments.

We judge ourselves much harder than anyone else ever would. Don generously taught me that day a mindfulness practice in a very easy, relaxed way.

He did not chastise me for being so hard on myself. He paused and allowed me to recognize that for myself. Then he kindly had me begin again, this time leading with Non-Judgment toward myself.

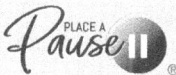

HOW DID IT GO?

I am inviting you to try this practice today!

Ask someone you know how their work is going?

Ask a friend or loved one how they are doing?

Mindfulness is a practice of compassion, so the intention you set, and your delivery are critical.

If they begin by beating themselves up about something they did or did not do, then I invite you to kindly ask them to pause and begin again. You can explain that first you would like to hear what is going right with the big project they are working on.

Would this work with your child when they return home from school, and you ask them how their day went? YES.

EXTRA CREDIT

I invite you to ask yourself right now, "How is your day going?" And begin with what is going well.

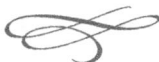

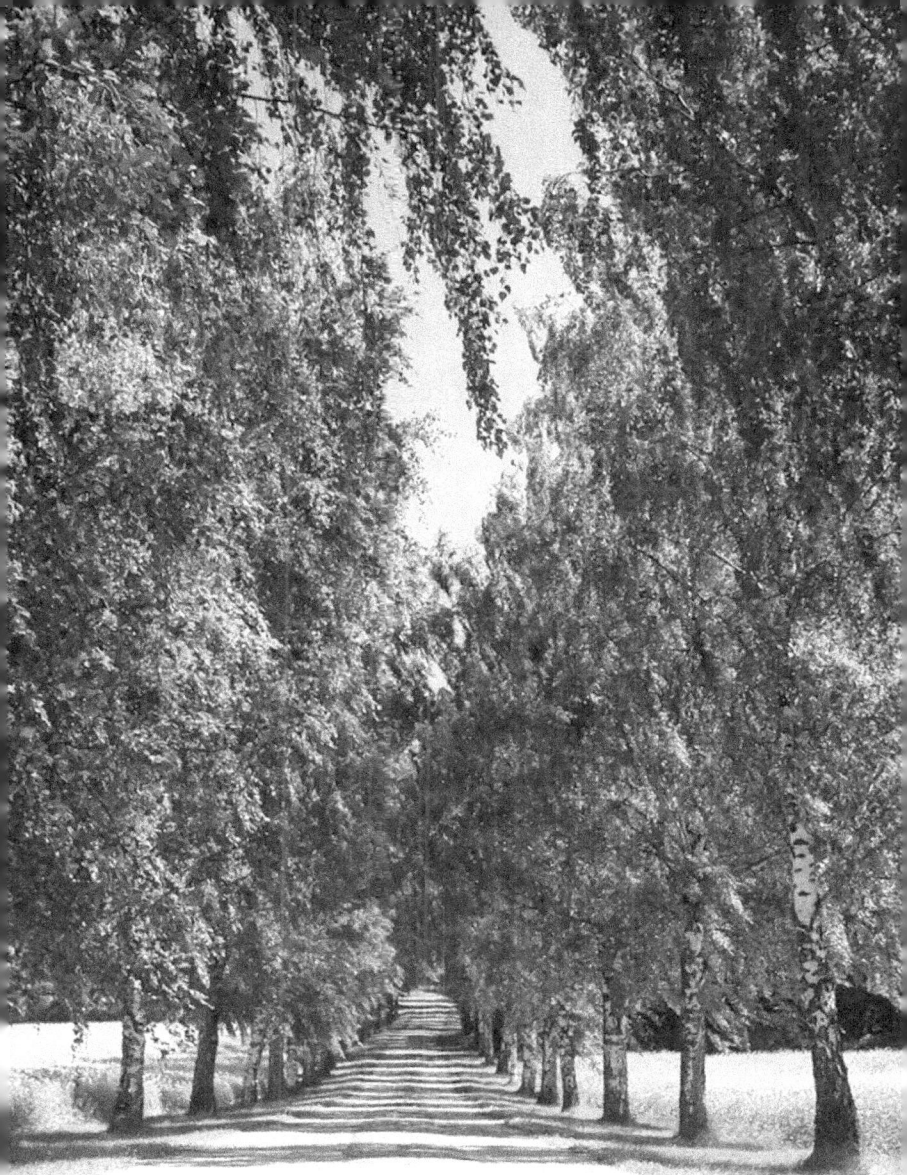

GRATITUDE

Gratitude

I am first sharing the following personal story because one of the most important indicators for a long life is one's ability to make new connections with people. After all, when one lives to an advanced age, they have lost many of the people they once loved.

I NEVER THOUGHT I WOULD FALL IN LOVE AGAIN

It was a big leap of faith for me when I moved out of my townhouse in the suburbs and into a condo located in a building with over 50 floors in Philadelphia.

I was involved in a long-distance relationship, and I didn't really have any friends in this city of over 1.5 million people. I simply trusted my intuition, which told me to follow my dream of living in the city.

One night shortly after I moved in, I was awoken at two o'clock when the fire alarm went off in the building. It was a loud siren followed by an announcement that said immediately move to the stairwell and wait for further instructions.

I was very scared because I was living on a floor that was above the reach of the highest fire truck ladder. I quickly threw on a pair of pants and a shirt, grabbed my pocketbook and phone, and got myself to the stairwell. Even though there were at least 30 people living on my floor of the building, I found myself standing there all alone.

And then the door opened and this little woman who was about 4' 9" tall came in wearing her flannel pajamas and a red raincoat. I was very nervous, but she was not really interested in hearing my small talk as I introduced myself as her new next-door neighbor. Finally, the siren stopped, and they told us we could return to our apartments.

The next day I ran in to my neighbor again, and this time we more formally introduced ourselves. I explained that I was very new to city living, and my new neighbor, Lillian, took me under her wing. I was so very grateful for her guidance on how to navigate living in the big city.

She wrote me a list of her favorite places to shop, her favorite places to go for different types of food, and where the best hardware store was located. Over the next several weeks we learned that we had so much in common. Neither one of us had ever been married; we were both registered nurses; we shared a religion. We both had one sister, though hers had passed, and we both grew up in the Philadelphia area. We would spend hours every night talking in the hallway, since Lillian was highly allergic to my cat.

Lillian was probably 87 years old when we first met, and within a very short period of time we became extremely close. When we would go out to lunch, I would tell people we were sisters. I could not ask for a more perfect neighbor. She once went out in an ice storm and fell getting onto the bus, and then fell getting off bus, just so she could surprise me with a mango that she bought from a local store and hung on my door knob.

One day after I had arranged her surprise 90th birthday party, she looked at me and said, "I never thought I would fall in love again."

Lillian knew I always wanted to write, so she told me I could never share the many (many!) wonderful doggerels I would find slid under my door when I came home from work.

I am so grateful I had the opportunity to meet and develop such an unexpected and loving relationship. I miss the wisdom she so freely shared with me, her laughter, her saucy jokes, but mostly her friendship.

ONE ROSE AT A TIME

There are very few rituals that I have ever honestly found meaning in. I'm admitting that now.

I never even understood the reason for funerals, until my own dear mother passed away almost 30 years ago. Then instantly I understood, since every person that day who hugged me, gave me the energy to continue. It was also then that I realized why we come together and celebrate the union of a couple getting married as well. I respected all the ceremonies I had attended, just experienced a much deeper understanding once I had the personal experience from the funeral of family and friends coming together.

After my mother passed away, I thought to myself, I'm going to try to never love anyone again so deeply so as to avoid this depth of pain I was experiencing from her loss.

And then time passed.

Buddy, a little kitten, came into my life three years after my mother's death. I broke my rule, and fell in love.

Buddy and I were together for almost 15 years, before he passed away. My brother-in-law sent me a dozen white roses in honor of Buddy. An interesting choice, since I never let flowers into my home because I was also afraid of one of my two cats injuring themselves somehow.

So, for the first time, I didn't hide the roses. I placed them in a vase and fortunately my five year old cat ignored them. However, every day I enjoyed them until they too died. And that is when I decided to pause.

I took the vase into the kitchen and stood next to the trash can. I took the first white rose and before tossing it away, decided to admire its beauty very closely, its softness, and wonderful scent…and then spontaneously I decided to thank Buddy for what he had brought into my life. Rose after rose I paused, and then thanked him; for coming to sleep next to me when I had lived alone, for the smell of his fur, for always coming to the front door to welcome me home no matter how sick he felt, for never running away from me, for the softness of his fur, and for letting me hold him when I needed at times to hold on…

After the sixth rose was placed in the trash and I paused, something happened.

It was as if Buddy now wanted to thank me. I had not expected this, but paused and continued.

Buddy began with rose number seven; thanking me for caring for him when he was sick, for rescuing him from the shelter, for going through so many different types of food when I couldn't find one he liked anymore, for letting him sleep on me, for keeping him safe, and for my smell and gentle touch.

I had never had a pet before Buddy, and had not cried this much since the loss of my own mother.

Sometimes after a loss it is normal to "contract" and to never want to love again. And with Buddy, I learned that love is indeed worth the pain of losing someone. He taught me to "expand."

Weeks passed before I could walk into a pet store again. When I did, I walked directly to the area with cats that needed to be adopted. I looked into their eyes as they sat in small metal cages hoping to be set free, and realized that on this planet, there will always be others who need our love. Always.

I could have easily picked up the bunch of roses and quickly tossed them in the trash that day. Like I said, I have never practiced any rituals before.

Though I am so grateful, that on that day, I was so present with my intention of wanting to honor my Buddy, that I paused and noticed…and remembered.

And fortunately, I had taken the time to have created all those memories, I now treasure, when spending time with him.

NO, THAT'S TOO MUCH MONEY!

Do you remember the last incredible person who served you in a restaurant? I surely do.

I was having lunch with a girlfriend and this waiter, who told us his name was Rob, was providing impeccable service. You know the type. Extra napkins provided before you ask for them. Dressing on the side automatically. Brings out more hot water for your tea when he notices your cup getting low.

Before I left, I thanked him and said I would be telling his manager how excellent the service was that he provided. I then handed him a ten-dollar bill, instead of the $8 tip which would have been 20%.

Rob replied, "No, that's too much!"

I was shocked, but made sure he took the money. He explained how grateful he was since he was having a very bad day. He was dealing with terrible headaches and had to take a leave of absence from his career path due to a death in his family. He was now going back to school to become a massage therapist so he could help others.

Rob had given us no indication that he was feeling unwell as he took such great care in serving us, ensuring we had a lovely lunch experience.

Everyone is dealing with something. Everyone.

YOU ARE HERE TO TAKE CARE OF YOURSELF

On the very first day of my teaching practicum to learn how to teach the Mindfulness Based Stress Reduction eight-week program, I learned an invaluable lesson for which I will always be grateful.

As I quietly sat there during our first group sitting meditation practice, I noticed the person next to me was sneezing and blowing her nose a few times.

At the conclusion of the practice, my teacher asked us one by one how we were currently feeling in our body. What did we notice? Most shared that they felt calm, peaceful, or sleepy.

I replied, "I was sending positive energy to the woman next to me who sounded like she wasn't feeling very well."

My teacher kindly replied, "Harriet, you are here to listen to yourself, how it feels in your body, and not to be caring about anyone else's needs right now."

My first day and already I thought I had messed up.

And that is why I'm so grateful I went through advanced training to learn how to teach mindfulness. It was critically important as a teacher for me to be able to hold my seat and trust that everyone present was taking care of themselves.

My role as a teacher was not to be fixing or praying for anyone during my sitting meditation practice. Later we were taught the Loving Kindness meditation practice, in which you specifically focus loving energy toward yourself and then others.

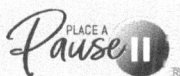

Place a Pause ⏸

FOR YOURSELF!

Take a moment right now and fully notice how it feels to be in your body... Noticing where your body is making contact with whatever you are sitting on... Feeling your weight on the back of your legs... Just resting in the moment...with no place to go and nothing to do for the next few minutes.

And when your mind wanders, as it surely will, just noticing that as if you were outside and saw a cloud drifting through the sky... Noticing your thoughts without judgment... And then escorting your attention right back to how it feels to be sitting.

Maybe even placing a hand right now on your abdomen and noticing your breathing with a fresh curiosity... How when you inhale your abdomen rises and when you exhale it just naturally falls back down.

Not needing to change or manipulate your breathing in any way... Just noticing it. Is it fast or slow? Is it deep or shallow? Maybe even noticing how at the end of every exhalation our bodies just naturally take a pause.

Noticing your in breath, how your clothing might gently move, how your ribs expand, followed by the out breath, and then maybe just resting in that pause. And watching how when your body is ready, it will automatically take that next in breath.

And remembering that this space is available for you to return to whenever you need it, just by placing a pause in your day.

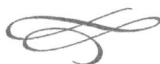

Consider the Financial Impact

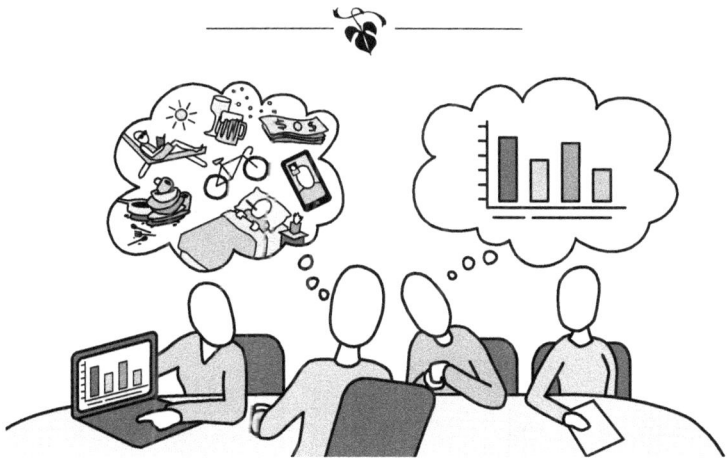

IS THERE AN ROI
(RETURN ON INVESTMENT)
TO MINDFULNESS?

My dear friend (we'll call him Brad to protect his privacy) looked me right in the eye and said, "Harriet, I talk with CEOs every day, and they couldn't care less if their staff is up all night and can't sleep. They are not thinking about their employees' stress."

I looked at Brad in amazement. It really hurt my heart, but I needed to hear it. So, I replied, "What if they knew I could quickly and easily teach their employees a practice that could impact their company's healthcare costs?"

"That," Brad continued, "they would surely be interested in."

I've had the honor of working with CEOs who are very concerned about the health of their employees.

And I frequently hear from HR leaders that the number one problem they are currently faced with is the mental wellbeing of the employees they support.

So, I respectfully ask you, "How much is this problem costing your company?"

As a nurse, I knew that 2020, 2021, and 2022 would be very stressful. I did my best to communicate this information and support every client, friend, and relative I knew. I shared my concern with my sister, who is a therapist.

She patiently listened to me and then replied, "This stress will continue for years because of the ongoing grief process."

She reminded me of all the different kinds of losses people have been through and will continue to need to process.

- The loss of loved ones and their limited funerals.
- The loss of celebrations that were dreamed about and planned for years. Weddings. Graduations. Vacations.

- The loss of good health as people struggle with long haul symptoms from the coronavirus.

- Even the simple joy of taking your newborn out in the stroller for some fresh air each day was stripped away from many first-time moms.

A mindfulness practice can decrease their stress.

Having healthy employees who are focused and able to complete the job they have been hired to do, safely and on time, can ultimately save your company money. Now, not later, is when you want to introduce a mindfulness practice into your life and into the lives of your colleagues and team members who are working so awfully hard for you, for your company, and for their families and friends.

Are you thinking, "I don't have time for this," or "We don't have time for a program right now."

How much is it costing you to have your employees out sick? How much productivity is lost when a member of your team shows up to your next meeting distracted and not really present? Isn't it finally time to learn another way to deal with all the challenges we now face?

To quote the valuation expert and author Dave Bookbinder, "The value of a business is a function of how well the financial capital and the intellectual capital are managed by the human capital. You'd better get the human capital part right."

ARE YOU SICK YET?

How are you feeling right now?

- Meeting all your business goals and objectives, your sales quotas?
- Family commitments taking up a lot of your time?
- The HOLIDAYS! Yes, they're coming up quickly too!

Okay, I'll stop there so you can sleep tonight.

SPOILER ALERT, as a nurse let me tell you how this plays out.

"I don't feel good, it must be...

- my allergies."
- a cold my child brought home from school."
- my sinuses; they always act up this time of year."
- my stomach; it has been acting weird."
- from when I hurt my back at the gym."
- that I need to get to the gym!"
- this season; it is always when I get migraines."

It does **NOT** have to be this way!

The mind and the body work together. Your body is listening to you. It can hear you say, "How am I ever going to get all of this done? I don't even look forward to the holidays anymore, or even the weekend."

I think we can all agree it is more socially acceptable to say, "I don't feel good," than to admit, "I have too much to do! I'm exhausted!" Or the latest version I now frequently hear, "I'm tired of adulting."

A mindfulness program is not complicated. You do not have to get up at 4:30 am and go to the gym or drag your tired self there at night. This is why I wrote this book, and speak on this topic at conferences, and teach programs internally for organizations.

And since Mindfulness is a practice of Non-Judgment, please do not judge yourself or others if any of this rings a bell.

You truly are doing the best you can!

Burnout is now a legitimate medical diagnosis, according to the International Classification of Diseases.[11] (ICD-11), the World Health Organization's handbook that guides medical providers in diagnosing diseases.

Per the handbook, doctors can diagnose someone with burnout if they present the following symptoms:

1. feelings of energy depletion or exhaustion

2. increased mental distance from one's job, or feelings of negativism or cynicism related to one's job

3. reduced professional efficacy

HOW TO LIVE YOUR DREAM!

Many years ago, after a conference session, I approached an internationally known scientist and writer, Jon Kabat-Zinn, the teacher who introduced me to the practice of mindfulness, for some advice. I was hoping he would share a colleague's name to help me move into a new career. Jon listened intently as I tried to boil down decades of my life and professional experience into five minutes.

His advice was simple. "Why not just put your big toe in the water?" He smiled and continued, "Just take one little step; try just one little thing."

I smiled in return, thanked him, and walked away confused because what I hoped for was a connection.

Looking back at that moment, I realize he gave me so much more. He gave me an honest answer about how to create the life I wanted to live. I contemplated the meaning of Jon's words for months. Just put my big toe in the water. Slowly – V...E...R...Y... S...L...O...W...L...Y – I started doing just that. I began to make choices, conscious choices, and pay attention to what would truly make me happy.

As Jon suggested, I started small. I was working as a training manager at a global pharmaceutical company and asked my manager if I could teach people a bit about mindfulness over lunch. Thankfully, she agreed, but suggested I keep it rather quiet. The first week, I had two people in the conference room.

The following week, there weren't enough chairs to accommodate the crowd!

I led that weekly 25-minute lunchtime program for over nine years, and taught over 5,000 of my colleagues. I was honored to be asked to present at the company's Rising Leader Program and invited to speak at their global leadership forum.

Mindfulness was never part of my job description. It was always something I did on the side as long as it didn't affect my job responsibilities. But eventually, I chose to change careers and "live my dream."

So now you know why I named my company Big Toe in the Water. It is my homage to Jon Kabat-Zinn, who taught me how to pay attention so as not to miss even one moment of my life.

If you have a dream or are confused or frustrated with where you are in your life, why not consider putting your big toe in the water?

TESTIMONIALS FROM REAL PEOPLE

Honestly, the only testimonial that matters is yours!

If you want to know if a mindfulness practice makes an impact, then I invite you to test drive it for yourself. Try it out. Kick the tires.

If you have any interest in what others have experienced, then feel free to check out my profile on LinkedIn and read some testimonials from real people who have experienced one of my mindfulness programs. https://www.linkedin.com/in/harriet-stein

Dear Reader,
I look at reviews before I purchase any item. Therefore, if you found this book valuable, I would appreciate you sharing your review online wherever you bought this book. Thank you!

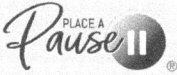

FOR A TEST DRIVE

You do not need to buy a journal; just find some paper or start a new note on your phone or computer, and write down how you feel right now in your body. What is your mood? List everything on your mind.

Now take a step back, and without judging them, and with an open mind and heart, become curious about the thoughts you have written down. Are they a mixture of present, past, and future items?

As you begin to practice what you have learned in this book, take the time to write down at least one sentence daily regarding what you are noticing about yourself.

Maybe you notice a lot of items in the past column, and that is just how it is right now, and not necessarily how it might be when you check in with yourself again in another hour or another day.

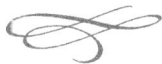

How to Make this Practice Stick!

An easy way to make this practice a part of your life, is to frequently bring your awareness to what you are thinking and doing.

One simple way to accomplish this is to set an appointment with yourself every hour. It can be as simple as a brief reminder on your phone, calendar, or watch.

When that reminder goes off, I invite you to ask yourself the most important question you will ever ask yourself, "Where am I?"

This will allow you to decide where you want to spend your most valuable time and attention.

Place a **Pause** ®

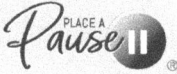

DURING TRANSITIONS THROUGHOUT YOUR DAY

Place a pause and practice:

- First thing in the morning, before you even get out of bed
- As you get dressed for your day
- Whenever you are moving from one activity to another
- Before, during, and after your meals
- When you experience a challenging text or call
- While waiting in line
- Getting in and out of your car
- On public transportation
- Prior to entering your home
- Before you go to sleep

Check-in with your Triangle of Awareness – notice your thoughts, the sensations in your body, and your current mood, moment by moment with non-judgment.

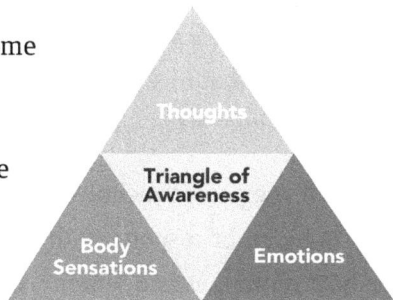

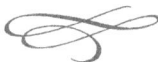

Thoughts

Triangle of Awareness

Body Sensations

Emotions

Conclusion: I'm Too Busy to Practice

Are you too busy to practice?

If you incorporate even small amounts of silence into your day, you'll have the space to think, be a better listener, and enable your mind to hear the wisdom that resides within you.

It's a choice. It's your choice whether or not to place a pause and listen for your inner wisdom and live a life with ease.

Are you too busy to bring mindfulness into your life? Or are you so busy that this might be the only way to provide yourself some relief from what you're dealing with?

We have the power to choose whether to succumb to the churn of reactivity, or respond with awareness about what is going on both around us and within us. We have the power to determine if we want to be lost in thought, frustrated with ourselves about past decisions, or needlessly worrying about the future.

Near the end of the Wizard of Oz the good witch Glinda appears, and (paraphrasing) Dorothy asks her, "Will you help me? Can you help me?"

And Glinda explains, "You don't need to be helped any longer. You always had the power to go back to Kansas."

And the scarecrow says, "What the…" Okay, maybe that's not exactly how he said it. He says something more like, "Why didn't you tell her before?"

And Glinda replies, "She wouldn't have believed me. She had to learn it for herself."

Can you now see how you've always had the power?

The power to let go of anger.

The power to stop regretting the past.

The power to stop worrying.

The power to create space to think and to be the best version of yourself.

It is as simple as pausing and paying attention to what is going on within you.

The power lies in leading our lives with awareness and knowing that the only moment that exists is the one you are living right now!

Be present for it!

Acknowledgements

My sister, Nancy Stein Hessenthaler, said to me in April of 2000, "I'm attending this one-day workshop with Jon Kabat-Zinn, and I think you'd enjoy it." That workshop, specifically Jon's teaching, changed my life forever, as I sat there interested, bored, exhausted, amused, and so many other emotions I had that day learning about and experiencing the practice of mindfulness. I am very grateful for all Jon has taught me over the years by attending his programs and through his writings.

I want to thank all the talented and generous teachers I've had the honor to learn from throughout my entire life.

I would not be able to teach had it not been for the excellent mindfulness teacher's program, I participated in led by Diane Reibel, who cofounded the Stress Reduction Program at Thomas Jefferson University in Philadelphia. Diane is the Director of the Myrna Brind Center for Mindfulness Marcus Institute of Integrative Health. Fortunately for me Donald McCown was still working at Jefferson and was instrumental in my teacher development before he left to become director of the center for contemplative studies at West Chester University of Pennsylvania. Diane and Don both remain my trusted teachers and now dear friends.

Theresa Hummel-Krallinger has been my unofficial mentor, business coach, trusted advisor, and shoulder to lean on. I honestly would not have a business without her. Our friendship began long before our business relationship, and I value it and her beyond words. She leads by example to squeeze the joy out of every day.

To all my clients who trusted me with their most prized possession, the hearts and minds of their colleagues, teams, leaders, and staff, I thank you. You helped me positively impact this world. And that's no small thing.

To Andria Flores who patiently read every word of this book, more than once, and is a joy to have as my editor, thank you. And I will embarrassingly admit I never understood the value of a proofreader until I experienced first-hand the expertise of Nancy Pendleton!

I would also like to thank my previous copy editors, Laurel Cavalluzzo and Erin Dalton, for the time we were able to work together.

I'm grateful for the many years of creative marketing and strategic designs, along with a massive amount of encouragement, provided by Julie Mueller and her team at jamgd. Cicely Combs, your ability to turn my words into illustrations is surely a gift. The works of art you created for me may not hang in galleries, but far more importantly, they are posted on the cubes and office walls of hundreds of people around the world as a way to refocus their lives.

I want to thank Debbie Phillips who acted as my trusted advisor and encouraged me to take on the development of a global train-the-trainer program, when I had never attempted anything so large before in my career. As the world shut down early in 2020, we jumped into action. It was her friendship, expertise, optimism, and strength that enabled me to create and launch a highly valued and meaningful program at the height of a global pandemic. The award-winning program continues to be taught globally, and as a nurse, to be able to make an impact by decreasing people's stress during the pandemic remains my most cherished achievement.

I wish I could list every friend and colleague, though I thank them all for the support they have given me throughout the years. If I listed them all, that would be an entire separate book.

I am also very fortunate to have been able to work with Lois Creamer, a talented 'speaker whisperer,' and author of *Book More Business*, another trusted advisor who immediately impacted my life with her ability to quickly bring me up to speed on the business end of speaking so I could share this invaluable practice at conferences and internally to organizations. Lois' colleague, Cathy Fyock, the business book strategist helped me from day one when I had no idea how to even begin this book. And then Cathy continued to support me with ways to market this book to ensure that the people I wrote it for would have access to reading it.

"Have you ever found yourself speaking, when much like a pilot you were trying to land a plane and ran out of runway?" I was watching a YouTube video of Michael Port, who with his wife Amy, founded Heroic Public Speaking (HPS), and he posed that question.

I thought to myself, "Exactly!"

I finally learned how to safely land that plane after working with Michael and Amy. And I became part of their HPS community, filled with talented and supportive speakers who I know will always have my back. As well as the incredible HPS team and editors (I'm talking about you AJ Harper, and your excellent book, "Write a Must-Read!").

Last, but surely not least, I want to thank my family. All of them!

Specifically, my husband, John Russell, who again and again, would kindly hold up the mirror of mindfulness in front of me whenever I grew weary or afraid. His generosity of spirit is resounding, when in life it is much easier to walk by or look away.

And to my uncle, Lee Schwartz, who has always been more like a brother to me. Whenever I have struggled, he has been there with a net, beginning when I was a child and throughout my entire life. I thank him for sharing all his knowledge with such humor and candor. His strength has seen me through my darkest days and his stories live in my heart.

I have already mentioned my sister who led me to teach Mindfulness by introducing me to Jon, though she has surely been the best 'older younger sister' anyone could be blessed to have. There are not enough words to express the gratitude I have for all that she means to my life. Much of what I teach, she has first taught me. Her strength and wisdom are only usurped by the size of her heart. I'm very grateful that the universe placed us on the same tram.

I was raised by two incredible people, my mother, Anne Stein, and my grandfather, Samuel Schwartz, who have now both passed. I'm grateful I had the opportunity to thank them when they were alive for making me the person, I am by the way they lived their lives.

And I thank you for buying this book, for reading all my stories and now maybe seeing life with a bit less judgment and a bit more love.

Now pause and go make a new memory!

Notes

———— ❧ ————

1. Mattei, M, (n.d.). Pete Carroll: Loud Practices & Quiet Minds in Seattle. MeetMindful. https://www.meetmindful. com/pete-carroll-loud-practices-quiet-minds/

2. TenGolf (May, 2021). Phil Mickelson: Winner 2021 PGA Championship Interview. YouTube. https://www.youtube. com/watch?v=fUpLXdnFOOY&t=790s

3. Big Ten Network, (December, 2022). "The Kid's Special." | Michigan QB J.J. McCarthy | Michigan Football | The Journey. YouTube. https://www.youtube.com/watch?v=fDEiAs-jsDA

4. Scipioni, J. (February, 2020). 2 things Serena Williams does every day to be productive. CNBC Make It. https://www.cnbc. com/2020/02/19/what-serena-williams-does-every-day-to-be-productive.html

5. Sonnentag, S. (2001). Work, recovery activities, and individual well-being: A diary study. Journal of Occupational Health Psychology, 6(3), 196–210. https://doi. org/10.1037/1076-8998.6.3.196

6. Park, Y., Fritz, C., & Jex, S. M. (2011). Relationships between work-home segmentation and psychological detachment from work: The role of communication technology use at home. Journal of Occupational Health Psychology, 16(4), 457–467. https://doi.org/10.1037/a0023594

7. European Cultural Centre (2022). Palazzo Mora 2022 Virtual Tour. Matterport. https://my.matterport.com/show/?m=D2BKg-WrZG1q

8. Marz, L. and Zorn, J. (March 2017). The Busier You Are, the More You Need Quiet Time. Harvard Business Review. https://hbr.org/2017/03/the-busier-you-are-the-more-you-need-quiet-time

9. McCarriston, S. (June, 2021) LOOK: Novak Djokovic hands young fan winning racket from the French Open, making for an adorable moment. CBS Sports. https://www.cbssports.com/tennis/news/look-novak-djokovic-hands-young-fan-winning-racket-from-the-french-open-making-for-an-adorable-moment/

10. Whitehead, N. (July, 2014). People would rather be electrically shocked than left alone with their thoughts. Science. https://www.science.org/content/article/people-would-rather-be-electrically-shocked-left-alone-their-thoughts-rev2

11. Burn-out an "occupational phenomenon": International Classification of Diseases. (May, 2019). World Health Organization. https://www.who.int/news/item/28-05-2019-burn-out-an-occupational-phenomenon-international-classification-of-diseases

Connect With Harriet

Having conducted and taught clinical research and witnessed the devastation that stress takes on our bodies, as well as our personal and professional lives, Harriet Stein understands the unique challenges that businesses face today, whether it be the need to lower healthcare costs, increase productivity, or boost morale. She knows the positive impact of teaching people, both employees and their leaders, how to decrease their stress and increase their performance. Injecting humor and science into her engaging programs, Harriet shows companies of all sizes how the power of leading with awareness strengthens organizations and creates healthy working environments.

Harriet is the creator of Take a Pause, an award-winning international mindfulness training program. During her tenure at a Fortune 50 global pharmaceutical company, she used her expertise and passion to directly instruct more than 5,000 worldwide employees on the practice of mindfulness through engaging presentations and at leadership summits. And she has extensive experience teaching mindfulness practices and strategies at Fortune 500 companies to improve corporate culture.

Her first teacher was Dr. Jon Kabat-Zinn, founder of the Mindfulness-Based Stress Reduction program. She completed extensive professional training at the Myrna Brind Center for Mindfulness at Thomas Jefferson University Hospital. This advanced training, interwoven with her background as a Registered Nurse and her Master of Science degree in Health Administration, is foundational to the compassion and purpose she brings to her mindfulness teaching and practice.

Whether it's a keynote, executive retreat, or a multi-week program, Harriet customizes the deliverable to meet her clients' needs. To schedule Harriet to speak or find out more about her programs, please contact her at www.HarrietStein.com.

Harriet speaks at conferences and internally for organizations, businesses, and colleges.

For information visit
www.HarrietStein.com

For mindfulness tips and to learn about upcoming public programs, go to
https://www.HarrietStein.com/PerfectAttendance

About the Author

Harriet has spent her career working with organizations and their most valuable resource—their people.

Her work in mindfulness yields bottom line results for her clients. Creator of an award-winning global mindfulness program, member of the National Speakers Association, as well as a registered nurse, inspirational teacher, and professional speaker, Harriet is passionate about speaking to organizations of all sizes.

Her advanced training and formal education, her passion for mindfulness, and her witty delivery endears Harriet to her audiences. Mixing research and science with levity and fun, her proven strategies demonstrate tangible ways to live in the present and be accessible, both professionally and personally.

Harriet lives in Pennsylvania with her husband and cat, Sunny. Though born at the Jersey shore, this is why sand will always remain in her shoes.

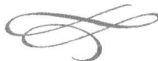